THE
PREMENSTRUAL
SYNDROME

THE PREMENSTRUAL SYNDROME

Proceedings of a workshop
held during the
Sixth International Congress of
Psychosomatic Obstetrics and Gynecology,
Berlin, September 1980

Edited by
Pieter A. van Keep and Wulf H. Utian
The editors were assisted by Pamela Freebody

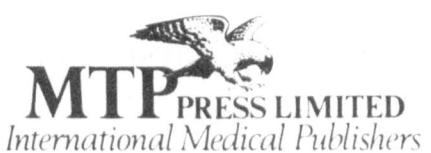
MTP PRESS LIMITED
International Medical Publishers

Published by
MTP Press Limited
Falcon House
Lancaster, England

Copyright © 1981 MTP Press Limited
Softcover reprint of the hardcover 1st edition 1981

First published 1981

ISBN-13:978-94-011-6257-9   e-ISBN-13:978-94-011-6255-5
DOI: 10.1007/978-94-011-6255-5

Contents

Principal participants 7

Preface
P. A. van Keep and W. H. Utian 9

1 Aetiology of premenstrual syndrome
J. B. Day and R. W. Taylor 11

2 The premenstrual syndrome – an epidemiological
and statistical exercise
P. A. van Keep and P. Lehert 31

3 Premenstrual syndrome – a holistic approach
*L. Dennerstein, C. Spencer-Gardner and
G. Burrows* 43

4 An appraisal of the role of progesterone in the
therapy of premenstrual syndrome
G. A. Sampson 51

5 An explorative study into the clinical effects of
dydrogesterone in the treatment of premenstrual
syndrome
J. R. Strecker 71

6 A double-blind, placebo-controlled, multi-centre
study of the efficacy of dydrogesterone
(Duphaston ʀ)
A. A. Haspels   81

Discussion A – between panel members
Chairman: W. H. Utian   93

Discussion B – between panel members and
members of the audience
Chairman: P. A. van Keep   105

Principal participants

J. B. Day
Department of Obstetrics and
  Gynaecology,
St Thomas' Hospital,
London SE1 7EH,
United Kingdom

L. Dennerstein
Department of Psychiatry,
University of Melbourne,
Clinical Sciences Block,
c/o PO Royal Melbourne Hospital,
Victoria 3050,
Australia

A. A. Haspels
Academisch Ziekenhuis Utrecht,
Universiteitskliniek voor Obstetrie
  en Gynaecologie,
Catharijnesingel 101,
Utrecht,
The Netherlands

P. A. van Keep
International Health Foundation,
Rue de Rhône 40,
1204 Genève,
Switzerland

G. A. Sampson
'Queenswood' Psychiatric Unit,
Middlewood Hospital,
PO Box 134,
Sheffield S6 1TP,
United Kingdom

J. R. Strecker
Universität Ulm,
Frauenklinik,
Prittwitzstrasse 43,
7900 Ulm/Donau,
West Germany

W. H. Utian
Department of Obstetrics-
  Gynecology,
The Mount Sinai Hospital,
University Circle,
Cleveland, OH 44106,
USA

7

Preface

Despite a plethora of theories, premenstrual syndrome (PMS) has remained an enigma. There has persisted in the literature a constant conflict as to the existence of the syndrome, a question as to whether it is one syndrome or several, and a debate as to whether the origin is psychic, somatic, or both. Advances in endocrinology, specifically in radioligand assays, allowing for accurate hormone measurements, have precipitated a more scientific evaluation of PMS in recent years. Nonetheless, difficulties have persisted in accumulating well-documented data because of the protean nature of the syndrome. Indeed, even at this time, the question of what requires measurement during the follicular phase of the cycle and the premenstrual phase remains unresolved, and is difficult to place in perspective.

In view of the persisting conflict between the organic and the psychological schools of thought, we, the editors of this book, considered the Sixth International Congress of Psychosomatic Obstetrics and Gynecology to be an ideal venue for a workshop in which both parties could be encouraged to participate. Towards this end, the organizing committee of the International Society of Psychosomatic Obstetrics and Gynecology (ISPOG) was approached, and their response was extremely encouraging. In this respect, we wish to record our thanks to the Scientific Committee of ISOPG for allowing this workshop to be organized under their auspices, but totally under our direction. We, in turn, stand responsible for the format and content of the workshop.

The current proceedings represent the outcome of the workshop, and we express our thanks to the invited participants and to the general discussants.

It is our overall conclusion that PMS must be regarded as an endocrinopathy. It should be emphasized, however, despite the increasing tendency to regard the syndrome as a somatic disease, that there are certainly psycho–social–cultural aspects that contribute to symptom formation. This multi-factorial causation of symptoms accounts for the variable responses to different forms of therapy, including the marked response to placebos.

In presenting these proceedings we hope that the contents will act both as a source of information to clinicians and as a catalyst for further in-depth research into all aspects of PMS. We do believe that PMS as an endocrinopathy has 'come of age' and is accordingly deserving of a place in the future, not only at psychosomatic meetings, but also at scientific endocrine conventions. The surface of this problem has only been scratched; a considerable amount of in-depth research remains an urgent necessity.

Pieter A. van Keep
Wulf H. Utian

January 1981

1
Aetiology of premenstrual syndrome

J. B. DAY and R. W. TAYLOR

INTRODUCTION

Over the past 5 years a large number of papers have been written on the subject of premenstrual syndrome (PMS). These have covered the scientific basis of the syndrome, as well as treatment. A great deal of information has been collected, but no clear underlying cause of the syndrome has been found, probably because multiple factors are implicated.

Several theories as to the aetiology of PMS have been put forward, but it has often proved difficult to learn much from papers on this subject, firstly because many of the theories advanced are based on studies involving too few patients, and secondly because the conclusions reached by one author are seldom confirmed by another.

There is one area of knowledge, however, in which definite advances have been made, and that concerns the hormonal changes which take place during the menstrual cycle. It is likely that this is an area where still further important information will be obtained in the future.

In this paper we first briefly consider the psychogenic background to the PMS; we then discuss the hormonal factors which appear to be implicated in the aetiology of this syndrome, the way in which hormonal changes during the menstrual cycle may produce PMS symptoms, and finally the actions of the various types of treatment currently available. On this last point, ideally all treatments should be measured against other drugs and against placebo in controlled surroundings, but when treating PMS one must take care that this control does not produce its own set of inaccuracies. There is now good evidence that in PMS the placebo effect of treatment as such is very strong.

Psychogenic background

It has been stated that PMS is an evolutionary syndrome (Rosseinsky and Hall, 1974), the changing moods, with hostility and aggression during the premenstruum, increasing the male's ardour while keeping him at a distance until the fertile period approaches – this fertile period coinciding with a peak of human female sexuality at mid-cycle (Adams *et al.*, 1978). This, in 1980, is probably an unrealistic theory. It is true, however, that for some women menstruation becomes an unnecessary intrusion into an already difficult life. Premenstrual tension, with its depression and irritability, may be a reflection of this. Paige (1971), confirming the work of Grant and Pryse-Davies (1968), found that despite the presence of menstruation women on combined or sequential oral contraceptives do not experience these cyclic mood changes. It seems, however, that today some women taking these preparations do experience PMS, a fact which may well be related to the lowering in recent years of the hormonal content of many of the contraceptive pills available.

Berry and McGuire (1972), using a questionnaire, related sexual role to cyclical symptoms and found no evidence that PMS symptoms were associated with psychosocial or psychosexual aspects of women's lives. Menstruating women, however, appear to have greater mood swings during their cycle than those who have had a hysterectomy (Beumont *et al.*, 1975).

If the complaint by women of their normal physiology is considered an abnormal response, then these women do indeed have a neurotic tendency, but Pennington (1957) found that 95% of women have premenstrual symptoms, thereby suggesting that PMS is intrinsic and physiological. The problem of relating PMS to neuroticism is well described by Clare (1977), who pointed out that the symptoms used to score neuroticism overlap heavily with those used to score PMS. Coppen and Kessel (1963) found a positive correlation between neuroticism and severe PMS in 500 patients randomly sampled; this may be a valid point, but we are no nearer answering the question of aetiology. It is also interesting to note that PMS occurs in the mentally retarded in whom frustration and emotional disturbances are rarely seen (Takayama, 1972). The findings of Kantero and Widholm (1971) suggest either a genetic element to the condition or a psychosomatic induction of the syndrome, since 63% of daughters of unaffected mothers are symptom-free, whereas 70% of the daughters of affected mothers are themselves PMS sufferers.

The psychogenic influences surrounding a woman during her menstrual cycle may adversely affect her psychologically, thereby increasing the magnitude of any existing problems. The occurrence of menstruation, the awareness of ovulation, and then premenstrual symptoms, may form a potential cycle of stress for any woman. The stress produced may well increase anxiety and depression during the premenstruum.

PMS, to some, is a major disturbance but one which is well-accepted. To relate 'neuroticism' to such people, when their problem is brought about by a biochemical change, seems unhelpful when discussing aetiology.

In summary, PMS for any individual will have a considerable input from the woman's personality, which in turn will be affected by her surroundings. The individual's stress may further exaggerate an inherent biochemical change.

Ovarian steroids

Frank in 1931 focused on an 'oestrogen excess' as a causative factor of PMS, and Israel (1938) thought it not an excess of oestrogen but a 'lack of progesterone antagonism'. Hormonal measurements in those times were all indirect, and Israel demonstrated an abnormal secretory phase by endometrial biopsy. He could not, however, understand why PMS was not seen in anovular cycles.

Other workers followed using indirect assessment of hormone function in the luteal phase, and all basically supported the idea that the progesterone to oestrogen ratio is low in PMS patients (Greene and Dalton, 1953; Rees, 1953; Morton, 1950).

The direct evidence of the phase of ovarian steroids comes from work by Bäckström and Carstensen (1974) and Munday (1977) who performed plasma estimations of progesterone and

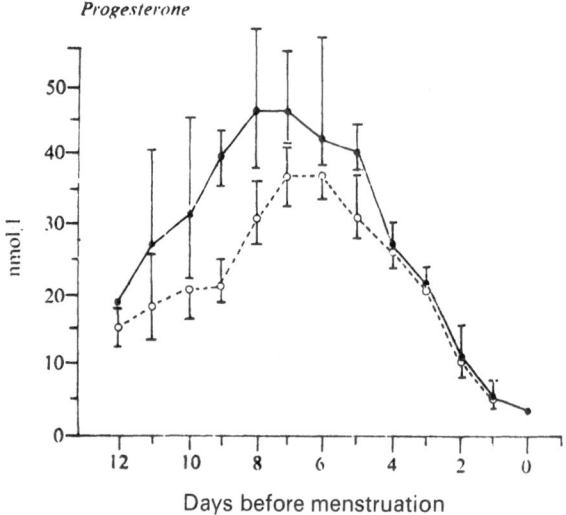

Figure 1 Logarithmic mean (± SEM) of plasma progesterone levels prior to menstruation in 20 women with premenstrual syndrome (o----o) and in ten control cycles (●——●). (Munday 1979. Reproduced with permission)

oestrogen or oestradiol, and it is these findings which form the basis of our present understanding. A trend has been found by these workers, both initially and more recently, but it should be pointed out that the daily fluctuations found by others have not always confirmed the findings of these two groups.

Bäckström and Carstensen (1974) compared daily steroids from eight women with no PMS with those of ten women with premenstrual anxiety and irritability. The progesterone levels in days 1–3 prior to menstruation were the same for both groups, but in days 4–10 premenstrually both oestrogen and progesterone were low in a small group with PMS. The oestrogen values rose to a peak above controls 4 days premenstrually, while progesterones continued to be low. There were no differences in LH values or in levels of the sex hormone binding globulin. FSH levels were higher in the PMS group 6–9 days premenstrually, after which they fell to the levels in control subjects.

Munday and her co-workers at St Thomas' Hospital in London found there to be lower progesterone levels in the PMS

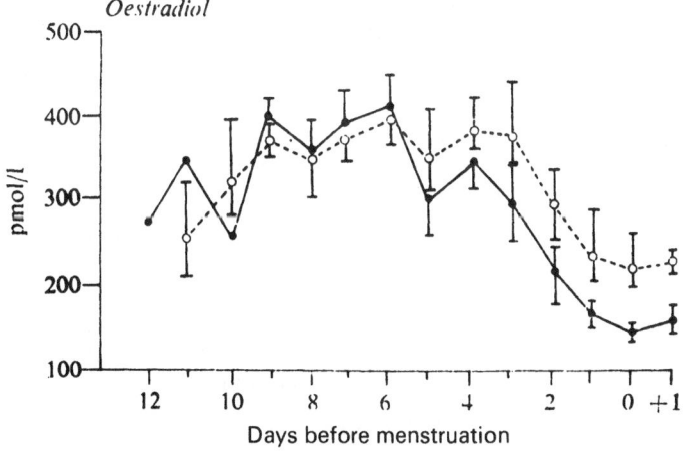

Figure 2 Logarithmic mean (± SEM) of plasma oestradiol levels prior to menstruation in 20 women with premenstrual syndrome (o– – – –o) and in ten control cycles (●——●). (Munday 1979. Reproduced with permission)

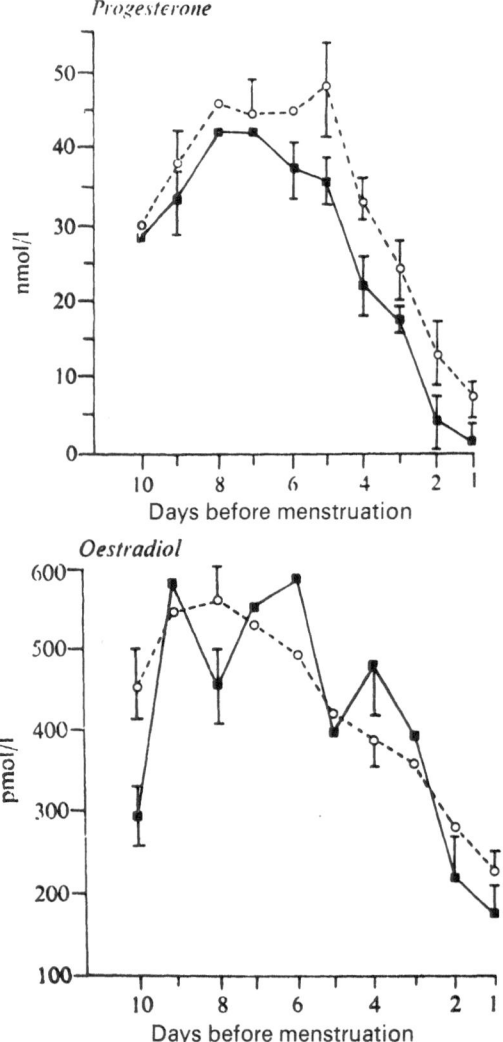

Figure 3 Daily mean (± SEM) plasma progesterone and oestradiol levels in ten control patients (■——■) compared with mean values for controls (○————○). (Munday, 1979. Reproduced with permission. The control data are those of Bäckström, who has kindly given permission for their reproduction here)

group at the mid-luteal phase from days 5–10 premenstrually (Figure 1). Munday concluded that after ovulation progesterone seemed impaired in the PMS group. The oestradiol levels were similar to those of the controls but were slightly higher in PMS patients after the mid-luteal peak of progesterone. A significant difference was shown from 4 days before menstruation until 1 day after it (Figure 2). The progesterone to oestradiol ratio was also calculated and found to be significantly higher in the controls for the last 8 days of the cycle. Munday's controls compared to those of Bäckström for plasma progesterone and oestradiol are shown in Figure 3. Smith (1975) found lowered progesterone levels, but no difference in plasma oestrogen.

It is only now that the significance of these first plasma results becomes apparent. They must be confirmed with as many as two samples per day in the follicular phase as well as in the luteal phase in patients with well-defined PMS and in controls.

Aldosterone and the renin angiotensin system

There is no evidence that aldosterone is a prime factor in the aetiology of PMS, although a premenstrual rise in plasma aldosterone in PMS patients was shown by Brush (1977) and by O'Brien et al. (1979). This rise, however, was no greater than in controls. The rise may be due to the progesterone levels of the luteal phase producing a natriuresis, followed by increased secretion of aldosterone to maintain homeostasis. The other possibility is that aldosterone metabolism may directly affect brain function. There is no evidence of this for aldosterone, but angiotensin appears to alter behaviour, central neurotransmitters and autonomic function in animals (Janowsky et al., 1973). It could, however, be postulated that an altered progesterone to aldosterone ratio may alter the stability of the RAA system and hence lead to symptoms of PMS. It is also interesting to note that several patients of O'Brien (1979), although complaining of bloatedness, showed no weight gain, suggesting that there are changes within the extra- and intra-vascular compartments. Aldosterone is a powerful antinatriuretic hormone, but so are oestrogens and antidiuretic hormone, and, to a lesser extent, prolactin and cortisol.

Prolactin

The place of prolactin is interesting, partly because the results available are conflicting. It is clear, however, that prolactin release is pulsatile (McNeilly and Chard, 1974), and that prolactin levels are not, therefore, constant.

Horrobin (1973) suggested that prolactin could be responsible both for the mental and for the physical symptoms of PMS. He was able to show that prolactin retains sodium and potassium.

Direct evidence in the form of serum measurements comes from Halbreich *et al.* (1976): four measurements made during the last 3 weeks of the cycle in 28 patients with PMS and in 21 controls showed that the PMS patients had a higher mean prolactin level and that their individual increases were also greater.

The use of bromocriptine has added further information on the place of prolactin. In controlled cross-over trials, Benedek-Jaszmann and Hearn-Sturtevant (1976) improved breast symptoms, oedema, weight gain and mood in patients attending an infertility clinic. Ghose and Coppen (1977), however, did not improve PMS patients by using bromocriptine; Andersen *et al.* (1977) improved mastodynia but none of their patients' other PMS symptoms. Five of the Andersen *et al.* patients had transient high levels of prolactin. Andersch *et al.* (1978) studied 20 PMS patients and 20 controls and found a luteal increase in prolactin; they also found that treatment with bromocriptine improved the PMS symptoms of breast discomfort and irritability.

The potential effect of prolactin on the length of the menstrual cycle should also be considered. Pronounced hyperprolactinaemia leads to amenorrhoea, but slightly raised levels produce a shortened luteal phase or are associated with this (Corenblum *et al.*, 1976; Benedek-Jaszmann and Hearn-Sturtevant, 1976). Two forms of inadequate luteal phase are described: a short luteal phase lasting less than 10 days with lowered steroid secretion (Strott *et al.*, 1970; Sherman and Korenman, 1974), and a defective luteal phase of normal length but with lowered steroid secretion (Pearce *et al.*, 1971; Dodson *et al.*, 1975). The aetiology of these defects is not known, but prolactin hypersecretion was implicated by Lenton *et al.* (1977) who noted slightly raised prolactin levels in the early follicular phase in women with a suspected, though not proven, inadequate luteal phase. Workers at St Thomas' Hospital found a raised prolactin level in association with a low progesterone level in PMS patients compared to controls (Brush, 1979) (Figure 4).

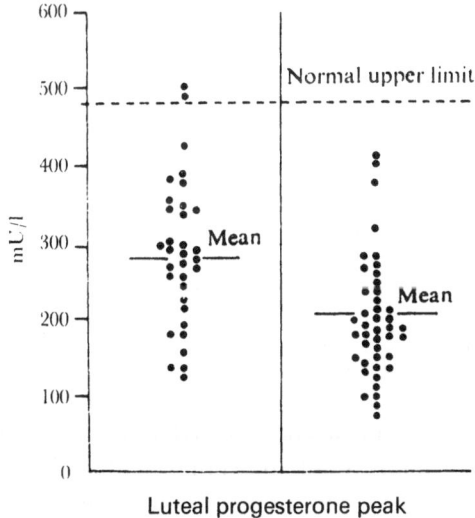

Figure 4 Comparison of serum prolactin levels in 33 premenstrual syndrome subjects with a 'low' progesterone curve (left panel) and in 42 subjects with a 'normal' progesterone curve

Precise interactions of prolactin with other hormones during the menstrual cycle are not known. Prolactin is known to inhibit the positive feedback of oestradiol on the LH peak at mid-cycle (Aono *et al.*, 1976; Glass *et al.*, 1975); the LHRH response from the pituitary in patients with hyperprolactinaemia is unaffected (Mortimer *et al.*, 1973; Zarate *et al.*, 1973), implying that the positive feedback of oestradiol to the hypothalamus is blocked in hyperprolactinaemia. Prolactin might also have a direct effect on the ovary (McNatty *et al.*, 1974).

The prolactin effect in the production of PMS may be via the lowering of progesterone and oestradiol levels during the luteal phase, or it may act directly on mineral and water metabolism. It may act directly on the breast, but not all hyperprolactinaemia patients develop galactorrhoea (Seppälä *et al.*, 1977).

Other theories on the aetiology of PMS

Hyperinsulinism in the premenstrual phase was suggested as a cause of PMS by Billig and Spaulding (1947). We now know that hypoglycaemia would cause a transient rise in prolactin.

An allergic response to steroids was suggested by Rogers (1962), who claimed successful treatment with minute quantities (0.1–1.0 μg) of pregnanediol injected subcutaneously.

Several vitamins have been thought to be implicated. The first mentioned was vitamin B (Biskind, 1943). More recently pyridoxine deficiency (vitamin B_6) has been suggested as a potential cause of the syndrome (Brush, 1977); in the form of pyridoxal-5-phosphate, vitamin B_6 is a co-factor in a number of the body's enzyme reactions. Particularly important is its place as a co-enzyme in the production of dopamine from tyrosine and of serotonin from tryptophan. At present there is no information regarding pyridoxal phosphate blood levels in PMS patients, though an assay has been described by Bhagavan *et al.* (1976).

A relative deficiency of vitamin B_6 has been suggested as a cause of depression in patients taking the combined oral contraceptive pill; this has been successfully treated with pyridoxine (Adams *et al.*, 1973, following an initial observation by Rose, 1969).

Treatment of PMS patients with pyridoxine was disappointing for Stokes and Mendels (1972), but Kerr (1977) and Day (1979) found it helpful to some extent. More controlled studies are required in this connection, together with assays of pyridoxal phosphate, though these may prove disappointing.

AN AETIOLOGICAL MODEL (Figure 5)

From the data available at present there is a definite suggestion that there are alterations in the progesterone and oestradiol levels in some PMS patients. This has the effect of producing a lower progesterone to oestradiol ratio during the last 7–10 days of the menstrual cycle, the progesterone levels being low in the early- and mid-luteal phase, while oestradiol levels are normal, the oestradiol levels then rising significantly 4 days premenstrually. Added to this is the evidence from Bäckström *et al.* (1976) that FSH levels are higher in the mid-luteal phase.

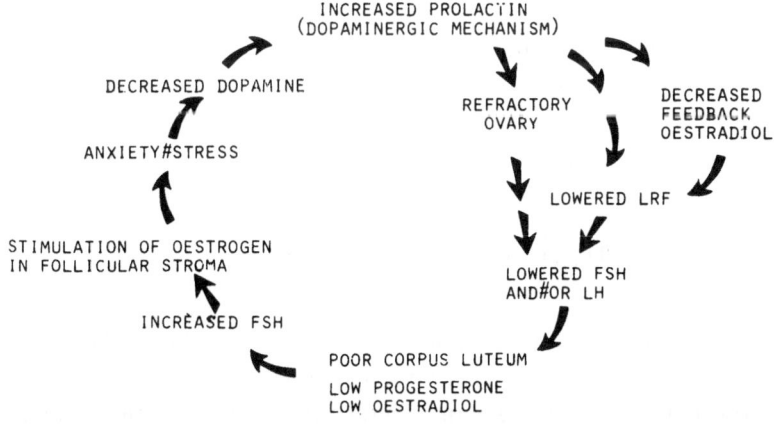

Figure 5 Aetiological model

21

Finally, the variability of prolactin must be included, with a tendency for raised levels in patients with PMS. A raised prolactin level early in the cycle, even if transient, due to stress or a hypothalamic factor, may lead to impaired follicular development and abnormal secretion of oestrogen and progesterone. The LH peak may not be affected, but a defective luteal phase may still follow. The abnormal follicle and altered level of oestrogen and progesterone would then allow a positive feedback to the pituitary and/or hypothalamus, and a luteal surge of FSH. In response to FSH the oestradiol levels may then start to rise towards the end of the luteal phase; a second LH surge does not occur, however, because of the presence of progesterone. Once established, the asynchronous cycle may continue with increasing stress factor induced by the cycle itself. This asynchronous potential of follicular development can be demonstrated in women by the number of follicles in the human ovary at different stages of development (Fowler *et al.*, 1977).

Mechanisms for an altered progesterone to oestradiol ratio are via:

(1) an alteration of the steroid pathway within the corpus luteum, or because of an absolute deficiency or imbalance of granulosa and/or of thecal cells;
(2) the effect of gonadotrophin producing an effect on the cells of the corpus luteum or on other ovarian components;
(3) a direct effect of prolactin on steroid steroidogenesis.

THE PRODUCTION OF SYMPTOMS

All the hormones mentioned so far have powerful effects on the movement of minerals and water within the body. What is difficult to know is whether it is a central change that produces the peripheral changes or whether it is a local action which produces them.

There is now good evidence that the gonadal steroids oestradiol and progesterone accumulate in the central nervous system, and that they affect brain metabolism and neural function. When injected into rats, ^{3}H progesterone is taken up very quickly by the cortex, sub-cortex, brain stem and cerebellum, but the radioactivity is lost more quickly from these areas than from the hypothalamus.

The general impression is that progesterone is tranquillizing and hypnotic, and that oestrogen tends to increase nervous activity; a lowering of the progesterone to oestradiol ratio could, therefore, be expected to lead to an increase in tension and irritability.

The contradictory evidence is that the progesterone to oestrogen ratio is at its lowest in the follicular phase, with no equivalent pre-ovulation syndrome. In view of this, individual levels are probably not important, but thresholds of action of any particular hormone are. It may be envisaged that hormone action will only produce an effect after interaction with other chemicals or with neurotransmitters. The pharmacological effects produced may be either to modify the response of a hormone on a receptor site or to actually alter the binding site availability.

The biogenic amines are probably mediating factors where hormones do not act quickly; the two main groups are the indoleamines, such as serotonin, which is responsible for serotonergic transmitter systems, and the catecholamines, such as dopamine and noradrenaline, which are involved, respectively, in cholinergic and noradrenergic systems.

In the future the link between these amines and the regulation of hypothalamic releasing factors will be an important area of research.

Regarding the somatic symptoms, these are best divided into (a) breast symptoms and (b) fluid retention symptoms. The breast symptoms probably occur as a direct result of an end-organ hormone imbalance, with prolactin featuring strongly.

The fluid retention symptoms, on the other hand, are probably a general reflection of an altered fluid transference between cells, and here the changes of progesterone to aldosterone, progesterone to oestradiol, and/or progesterone to prolactin ratios are important.

THE MODE OF ACTION OF TREATMENTS

Progesterone and progestogens

Firstly, some progestogens promote symptoms of their own, a particular example being norethisterone with its powerful water-retaining characteristics. The efficacy of natural progesterone is difficult to explain, as it is unlikely to be related to the making up of a deficiency and thereby to improving, for example, the progesterone to oestradiol ratio.

We have had good experience with dydrogesterone, an orally administered progestogen which is well-tolerated by patients. We have found it particularly beneficial in connection with depression, anxiety and irritability, improvements which probably occur as a result of a central effect on the areas of the cortex producing changes of mood. We have found it less useful for the physical symptoms of PMS. Some of our recent studies have suggested that the progesterone level during the luteal phase is actually reduced in patients taking dydrogesterone. Other studies, however, have not found this to be so, a fact which further exemplifies how difficult it is to interpret isolated hormone levels in this syndrome.

Aldosterone inhibitor

The diuretic spironolactone should, through its anti-aldosterone action, release body fluid. This it does, and patients suffering premenstrual oedema find it very useful. The oedema does, however, return as soon as the administration of spironolactone is stopped, suggesting that its action is almost entirely within the kidney. A potential benefit of spironolactone is its progesterone-raising effect, probably via the adrenals. This may produce an overall improvement of the syndrome. A dydrogesterone/spironolactone preparation started just prior to mid-cycle would be an interesting thought if the syndrome is severe. It may be, however, that the two compounds would competitively block each other

Dopamine

Bromocriptine has had disappointing results except for its effect on mastodynia and mastalgia, a local action. Its lack of effect on other symptoms makes one inclined to think that the extra dopamine provided is unnecessary; it does not, for instance, 'raise' neurotransmission, improve mood, etc. If it could be shown that a patient had a dopamine shortage, bromocriptine may be effective for the treatment of the whole syndrome.

Antigonadotrophin

Danazol is a drug which is still under-evaluated as far as PMS is concerned. It produces a dramatic response in some patients, but it is difficult to predict in which ones. Small doses of danazol may well, through the changes it produces in the hypothalamus, be able to re-programme the timing of FSH release, the response to oestradiol, the LH surge, etc., and so actually stop the symptoms of PMS occurring. Clinical trials with this substance are needed.

Pyridoxine

There is no evidence that vitamin B_6 deficiency occurs as a result of dietary deficiency in northern European countries. This being so, vitamin B_6 replacement is illogical, unless it can be shown that it centrally blocks other symptom-producing transmitter substances. At this stage it is our feeling that the effects of pyridoxine in patients suffering PMS are those of a placebo.

Monamine oxidase inhibitors

These have been widely used with good effects in patients suffering depressive illnesses, but there are only a small number of PMS sufferers who would benefit from them. It is difficult to know how they produce their beneficial effects; it could be by permitting the accumulation of selected amines, or by protection from the metabolism of certain amines, or it may be that they act by maintaining amine levels in an area of homeostasis, such as the hypothalamus.

Placebo effect

Finally, it must be said that the placebo aspect is certainly one of the most effective parts of treatment, and although severe symptoms may not be improved dramatically there will often be some amelioration. The mere fact that a patient discusses the problem with her doctor, and receives sympathetic support, may well cause the stress factor to be palliated, and physiology at the hypothalamic level to return to normal.

References

Adams, D. B., Gold, A. R. and Burt, A. D. (1978). Rise in female initiated sexual activity at ovulation and its suppression by oral contraceptives. *New Engl. J. Med.*, **229**, 1145

Adams, P. W., Rose, D. P., Folkard, J., Wynn, V., Seed, M. and Strong, R. (1973). Effect of pyridoxine hydrochloride (vitamin B_6) upon depression associated with oral contraception. *Lancet*, **1**, 897

Andersch, B., Hahn, L., Wendestam, C., Öhman, R. and Abrahamsson, L. (1978). Treatment of premenstrual tension syndrome with bromocriptine. *Acta Endocrinol.*, **88** (Suppl. 216), 165

Andersen, A. N., Larsen, J. F., Steenstrup, O. R., Svendstrup, B. and Nielsen, J. (1977). Effect of bromocriptine on the premenstrual syndrome. A double-blind clinical trial. *Br. J. Obstet. Gynaecol.*, **84**, 370

Aono, T., Miyake, A., Shioji, T., Kinugasa, T., Onishi, T. and Kurachi, K. (1976). Impaired LH release following exogenous estrogen administration in patients with amenorrhea galactorrhea syndrome. *J. Clin. Endocrinol.*, **42**, 696

Bäckström, T. and Carstensen, H. (1974). Estrogen and progesterone in plasma in relation to premenstrual tension. *J. Steroid Biochem.*, **5**, 257

Bäckström, T., Wide, L., Södergård, R. and Carstensen, H. (1976). FSH, LH, Te-BG-capacity, estrogen and progesterone in women with premenstrual tension during the luteal phase. *J. Steroid Biochem.*, **7**, 473

Benedek-Jaszmann, L. J. and Hearn-Sturtevant, M. D. (1976). Premenstrual tension and functional infertility. *Lancet*, **1**, 1095

Berry, C. and McGuire, F. L. (1972). Menstrual distress and acceptance of sexual role. *Am. J. Obstet. Gynecol.*, **114**, 83

Beumont, P. J. V., Richards, D. H. and Gelder, M. G. (1975). A study of minor psychiatric and physical symptoms during the menstrual cycle. *Br. J. Psychiatry*, **126**, 431

Bhagavan, H. N., Koogler, J. M. and Coursin, D. B. (1976). Enzymatic microassay of pyridoxal-5′-phosphate using L-tyrosine apo-decarboxylase and L-(1-^{14}C) tyrosine. *Int. J. Vitam. Nutr. Res.*, **46**, 160

Billig, H. E. Jr. and Spaulding, C. A. Jr. (1947). Hyperinsulinism of menses. *Ind. Med.*, **16**, 336

Biskind, M. S. (1943). Nutritional deficiency in the etiology of menorrhagia, metrorrhagia, cystic mastitis and premenstrual tension; treatment with vitamin B complex. *J. Clin. Endocrinol.*, **3**, 227

Brush, M. G. (1977). The possible mechanisms causing the premenstrual tension syndrome. *Curr. Med. Res. Opin.*, **4** (Suppl. 4), 9

Brush, M. G. (1979). Endocrine and other biochemical factors in the aetiology of the premenstrual syndrome. *Curr. Med. Res. Opin.*, **6** (Suppl. 5), 19

Clare, A. W. (1977). Psychological profiles of women complaining of premenstrual symptoms. *Curr. Med. Res. Opin.*, **4** (Suppl. 4), 23

Coppen, A. and Kessel, N. (1963). Menstruation and personality. *Br. J. Psychiatry*, **109**, 711

Corenblum, B., Pairaudeau, N. and Shewchuk, A. B. (1976). Prolactin hypersecretion and short luteal phase defects. *Obstet. Gynecol.*, **47**, 486

Day, J. B. (1979). Clinical trials in the premenstrual syndrome. *Curr. Med. Res. Opin.*, **6** (Suppl. 6), 40

Dodson, K. S., MacNaughton, M. C. and Coutts, J. R. T. (1975). Infertility in women with apparently ovulatory cycles. I. Comparison of their plasma sex steroid and gonadotrophin profiles with those in the normal cycle. *Br. J. Obstet. Gynaecol.*, **82**, 615

Fowler, R. E., Chan, S. T., Walters, D. E., Edwards, R. G. and Steptoe, P. C. (1977). Steroidogenesis in human follicles approaching ovulation as judged from assays of follicular fluid. *J. Endocrinol.*, **72** (3), 259

Frank, R. T. (1931). The hormonal causes of premenstrual tension. *Arch. Neurol. Psychiatry (Chic.)*, **26**, 1053

Ghose, K. and Coppen, A. (1977). Bromocriptine and premenstrual syndrome: controlled study. *Br. Med. J.*, **1**, 147

Glass, M. R., Shaw, R. W., Butt, W. R., Logan Edwards, R. and London, D. R. (1975). An abnormality of oestrogen feedback in amenorrhoea–

galactorrhoea. *Br. Med. J.*, **3**, 274

Grant, E. C. G. and Pryse-Davies, J. (1968). Effect of oral contraceptives on depressive mood changes and on endometrial monamine oxidase and phosphatases. *Br. Med. J.*, **3**, 777

Greene, R. and Dalton, K. (1953). The premenstrual syndrome. *Br. Med. J.*, **1**, 1007

Halbreich, U., Ben-David, M., Assael, M. and Bornstein, R. (1976). Serum-prolactin in women with premenstrual syndrome. *Lancet*, **2**, 654

Horrobin, D. F. (1973). *Prolactin: Physiology and Clinical Significance* (Lancaster: MTP)

Israel, S. L. (1938). Premenstrual tension. *J. Am. Med. Assoc.*, **110**, 1721

Janowsky, D. S., Berens, S. C. and Davis, J. M. (1973). Correlations between mood, weight and electrolytes during the menstrual cycle: a renin–angiotensin–aldosterone hypothesis of premenstrual tension. *Psychosom. Med.*, **35**, 143

Kantero, R. L. and Widholm, O. (1971). Correlations of menstrual traits between adolescent girls and their mothers. *Acta Obstet. Gynecol. Scand.*, **14** (Suppl. 14), 30

Kerr, G. D. (1977). The management of the premenstrual syndrome. *Curr. Med. Res. Opin.*, **4** (Suppl. 4), 29

Lenton, E. A., Sobowale, O. S. and Cooke, I. D. (1977). Prolactin concentrations in ovulatory but infertile women: treatment with bromocriptine. *Br. Med. J.*, **2**, 1179

McNatty, K. P., Sawers, R. S. and McNeilly, A. S. (1974). A possible role for prolactin in control of steroid production by the human Graafian follicle. *Nature*, **250**, 653

McNeilly, A. S. and Chard, T. (1974). Circulating levels of prolactin during the menstrual cycle. *Clin. Endocrinol.*, **3**, 105

Mortimer, C. H., Besser, G. M., McNeilly, A. S., Marshall, J. C., Harsoulis, P., Tunbridge, W. M. G., Gomez-Pan, A. and Hall, R. (1973). Luteinizing hormone and follicle stimulating hormone tests in patients with hypothalamic–pituitary–gonadal dysfunction. *Br. Med. J.*, **4**, 73

Morton, J. H. (1950). Premenstrual tension. *Am. J. Obstet. Gynecol.*, **60**, 343

Munday, M. (1977). Hormone levels in severe premenstrual tension. *Curr. Med. Res. Opin.*, **4** (Suppl. 4), 16

Munday, M. R. (1979). Endocrine studies in the premenstrual syndrome. Ph.D. Thesis, University of London, UK

O'Brien, P. M. S., Craven, D., Selby, C. and Symonds, E. M. (1979). Treatment of premenstrual syndrome by spironolactone. *Br. J. Obstet. Gynaecol.*, **86**, 142

Paige, K. E. (1971). Effects of oral contraceptives on affective fluctuations associated with the menstrual cycle. *Psychosom. Med.*, **33**, 515

Pearce, M. A., Fahmy, D., Morgan, C., Evans, C., Groom, G., Boyns, A. R. and Cooke, I. D. (1971). Hormonal changes in patients with defective luteal phases. *J. Endocrinol.*, **51**, 24

Pennington, V. M. (1957). Meprobromate (Miltown) in premenstrual tension. *J. Am. Med. Assoc.*, **164**, 638

Rees, L. (1953). The premenstrual tension syndrome and its treatment. *Br. Med. J.*, **1**, 1014

Rogers, W. C. (1962). The role of endocrine allergy in the production of premenstrual tension. *West. J. Surg. Obstet. Gynaecol.*, **70**, 100

Rose, D. P. (1969). Oral contraceptives and depression. *Lancet*, **2**, 321

Rosseinsky, D. R. and Hall, P. G. (1974). An evolutionary theory of premenstrual tension. *Lancet*, **2**, 1024

Seppälä, M., Lehtovirta, P. and Ranta, T. (1977). Discordant patterns of hyperprolactinaemia and galactorrhoea in secondary amenorrhoea. *Acta Endocrinol. (Kbh)*, **86**, 457

Sherman, B. M. and Korenman, S. G. (1974). Measurement of plasma LH, FSH, oestradiol and progesterone in disorders of the human menstrual cycle: the short luteal phase. *J. Clin. Endocrinol.*, **38**, 89

Smith, S. L. (1975). Mood and the menstrual cycle. In Sacher, E. (ed.) *Topics in Psychoendocrinology*, pp. 19–58 (New York: Grune and Stratton)

Stokes, J. and Mendels, J. (1972). Pyridoxine and premenstrual tension. *Lancet*, **1**, 1177

Strott, C. A., Cargille, C. M., Ross, G. T. and Lipsett, M. B. (1970). The short luteal phase. *J. Clin. Endocrinol.*, **30**, 246

Takayama, T. (1972). A clinical study of premenstrual syndrome. In Morris, N. (ed.) *Psychosomatic Medicine in Obstetrics and Gynaecology*, p. 596 (Basel: Karger)

Taylor, R. W. and James, C. E. (1979). The clinician's view of patients with premenstrual syndrome. *Curr. Med. Res. Opin.*, **6** (Suppl. 5), 46

Zarate, A., Jacobs, L. S., Canales, E. S., Schally, A. V., de la Cruz, A., Soria, J. and Daughaday, W. H. (1973). Functional evaluation of pituitary reserve in patients with amenorrhoea–galactorrhoea syndrome utilizing luteinizing-hormone–releasing hormone. *J. Clin. Endocrinol.*, **37**, 855

2
The premenstrual syndrome – an epidemiological and statistical exercise

P. A. VAN KEEP and P. LEHERT

INTRODUCTION

Premenstrual syndrome is the collective name given to the problems which occur during the 2-week period before menstruation, and which are considered to be a prelude to menstruation. The list of symptoms regarded as being part of this syndrome is long and varied.

It is somewhat strange when one considers how many women appear to suffer from this phenomenon that more precise knowledge as to the extent of the problem is not available. Most of the few reports which have appeared on the subject have been in connection with studies conducted in very selected groups, and the figures relating to the incidence of the problem have varied considerably (Table 1).

It is strange too that the premenstrual syndrome, first described by Frank in 1931, is still today so vaguely defined. This fact also makes the various studies and reports difficult to compare. Premenstrual syndrome, as it is 'defined' at present, seems to differ considerably from one woman to another, which sometimes makes it difficult for a woman and for her doctor to recognize a particular problem as being part of this syndrome (Dalton, 1980). The matter is further complicated by the fact that the duration of the symptoms and their severity also appear to vary enormously. Many women experience their premenstrual symptoms for 2 or 3 days, but some regularly experience them for a week or longer, and whilst some women see these symptoms as little more than a quickly passing sign that menstruation is on its way, others are incapacitated to the extent that it is impossible for them to continue with their normal daily routines.

Table 1 Studies reporting the incidence of premenstrual syndrome (PMS)

Authors	Year	Group	Number	% with PMS
Bickers and Wood	1951	Factory workers (USA)	± 1500	36
Morton et al.	1953	Female prisoners (USA)	249	51
Kessel and Coppen	1963	GP practices (UK)	500	25
Sutherland and Stewart	1965	Hospital personnel and students (UK)	150	33
Herschberg	1966	Gynaecology patients (France)	5000	32
Wetzel et al.	1975	Students (USA)	589	40
Clare	1977	GP practices (UK)	521	75
van Keep and Haspels	1979	National probability sample (The Netherlands)	1493	47

It is important to obtain more insight into the frequency of premenstrual syndrome in the female population as a whole, because only then shall we understand how far this is a health problem. Epidemiological studies may also provide insight into the type of woman who is particularly prone to premenstrual syndrome, and may therefore help the clinician to recognize a patient.

It was against this background that the study reported in the present paper was undertaken. The statistical exercise was conducted on data obtained by the International Health Foundation during a study in France in 1978–9 (International Health Foundation, 1979). A few of the data from the survey are repeated here in order to explain the background to the exercise.

THE STUDY

The study was a postal one conducted in France with the help of Sofres Médical, the medical branch of a national opinion poll company, in December 1978 and January 1979. It involved 2501 women between the ages of 15 and 50 from all parts of the country. In order to obtain the desired sample size it was necessary to send out 3600 questionnaires. The return rate, therefore, was 69% (a rate which would possibly have been higher had the survey been conducted at a less busy time of year).

The questionnaire contained 39 questions, and great emphasis was laid on the fact that the symptoms being discussed were those occurring during the 2 weeks *before* menstruation. Twenty-five possible symptoms were listed in alphabetical order. They were:

Back-ache, kidney ache
Clumsiness, proneness to accidents
Cold sweats
Difficulty in concentrating and in remembering things
Dizziness, a feeling of being not quite well
Eye or sight problems
General 'out-of-sorts' feeling
Headaches
Hot flushes
Indecision, inefficiency
Insomnia
Moodiness, irritability, aggressiveness

Muscle stiffness
Ovarian pains
Painful, heavy legs
Painful, swollen, tender breasts
Pains in the pelvic area
Sickness, nausea
Skin problems (irritations, blotchiness)
Sleepiness, lethargy
Stomach ache
Tearfulness, depression
Tenseness, general uneasiness
Tiredness, general weakness
Weight-gain, puffiness

A space was also left in which the respondents could add other symptoms which they felt to be part of the premenstrual syndrome. Thirty-five women did so, but none of the symptoms added featured more than two or three times, so it is felt that the above list can probably be regarded as a fairly comprehensive one, at least as far as the lay public is concerned.

Of the 2501 women who completed the questionnaire, 943 (38%) said that they experienced premenstrual pains or symptoms every month. A further 684 (27%) said that they experienced them from time to time, and 290 (12%) said that they experienced them occasionally. Thus, 77% of the 2501 women taking part in this survey reported that they experienced premenstrual symptoms. In reply to a later question, only 354 (14%) of the 2501 respondents said that they had never experienced such symptoms.

Two factors are probably involved in the moving of a premenstrual symptom into the category of a premenstrual complaint or problem: (a) the time it lasts, and (b) its severity. In this study the first factor was covered simply by asking the respondents to indicate the number of days on which they usually had the symptom; the second was covered by asking them to indicate if each symptom troubled them a little, moderately or very much. The most frequently experienced symptoms, together with the number and percentage of women usually experiencing each of the problems for 7 days or more, and the number and percentage of women troubled 'very much' by each problem, are given in Table 2. The incidence of the less extensively experienced symptoms is summarized in the footnote.

Table 2 Number of women experiencing premenstrual symptoms, those usually experiencing such problems for 7 or more days, and those being troubled by them 'very much'. The percentage calculations are based on all 2501 respondents

	Women experiencing the premenstrual symptom		Women usually experiencing the symptom for 7+ days		Women being troubled 'very much' by the symptom	
	No.	%	No.	%	No.	%
Moodiness, irritability, aggressiveness	926	37	180	7	220	9
Painful, swollen, tender breasts	829	33	291	12	147	6
Back-ache, kidney ache	773	31	91	4	193	8
Pains in the pelvic area	771	31	77	3	206	8
Ovarian pains	643	26	73	3	176	7
Tiredness, general weakness	630	25	137	5	124	5
Weight-gain, puffiness	594	24	176	7	131	5
Painful, heavy legs	470	19	93	4	104	4
Tearfulness, depression	461	18	78	4	115	5
Tenseness, general uneasiness	451	18	111	4	116	7
Headaches	428	17	34	1	166	7

The following symptoms were also mentioned: muscle stiffness (13%), general 'out-of-sorts' feeling (12%), skin problems (irritations, blotchiness) (11%), hot flushes (11%), insomnia (8%), sickness, nausea (7%), difficulty in concentrating and in remembering things (5%), sleepiness, lethargy (5%), dizziness, a feeling of being not quite well (6%), stomach ache (3%), clumsiness, proneness to accidents (3%), eye or sight problems (3%), indecision, inefficiency (2%), cold sweats (2%)

An analysis of the data showed there to be three groups of women with a particular tendency to experience premenstrual symptoms:

(a) women who have, or who have had, children, as opposed to those who have not;
(b) women with irregular menstrual cycles, as opposed to those with regular cycles (the interpretation of 'irregular' and 'regular' was left to the respondents themselves);
(c) women with menstrual bleedings usually lasting 7 or more days, as opposed to women with a shorter period of menstruation.

The two groups of women, those with premenstrual syndrome and those without, did not differ significantly from each other as far as any of the other variables were concerned – such as age, education, socio-economic standing and marital status.

THE STATISTICAL EXERCISE

The statistical exercise was undertaken in order to see if the data obtained in France could in any way suggest why some women experience one premenstrual problem whilst others experience different ones.

For this exercise it was necessary to reduce the number of symptoms studied. This was done by grouping symptoms together, the clustering being done on 'clinical', rather arbitrary, grounds. Five groups of symptoms were thus arrived at:

D1 – skin problems (one symptom)
D2 – aches and pains (three)
D3 – symptoms related to water retention (three)
D4 – tenseness, general uneasiness, and fatigue (two)
D5 – 'nervous' symptoms (three).

It was then necessary to calculate a score for each woman in respect of each of these groups of symptoms. This was done by multiplying each complaint first by the number of days on which it was normally experienced, and then by the degree to which it was troubling, one for little, two for moderately, three for very much.

The next stage, and the main part of the exercise, was to fix the position of each woman in a five-dimensional space, each of the dimensions being governed by one of the groups of symptoms.

The result was the emergence of three very distinct and separate groups of women, outside of which very few were to be found.

Group A was governed primarily by D3 (symptoms related to water retention) and secondarily by D4 (general uneasiness and fatigue), all other symptoms being far less important (Table 3).

Group B was governed by D5 ('nervous' symptoms). The water retention symptoms (D3) and aches and pains (D2) were moderately important, but far less so.

Group C was governed by D2 (aches and pains), with D5 ('nervous' symptoms) playing a secondary and far less important role.

Table 3   Co-ordinates of the centres of gravity of the three groups

Group	D1	D2	D3	D4	D5	No. women	%
A	0.046	0.059	*0.572*	*0.330*	0.090	410	31.6
B	0.039	0.109	0.148	0.088	*0.624*	554	42.8
C	0.033	*0.771*	0.026	0.033	0.157	331	25.6

D1, skin problems, did not feature predominantly in any group. An analysis of the women who suffered skin problems showed that this was primarily a complaint of women over the age of 48; one wonders if this is not, in fact, a climacteric symptom rather than a premenstrual one. This is purely a matter of conjecture, however.

The next question was: Are there any explanations in the data available which might 'explain' why a woman is in one group as opposed to another, or rather, given the nature of the data available, are there any factors which dominate in any of the groups which might indicate the likelihood of a woman being in that group as opposed to any of the others? The only factors available were:

(a) socio-demographic factors: age, profession, husband's profession, parity, socio-economic standing, area of residence;

(b) physiological factors: length of menstrual cycle, duration of menstrual bleeding, cycle regularity, contraceptive use.

A segmentation analysis (Williams and Lambert, 1966) was used for this part of the exercise, and the analysis was based on 1064 respondents, all those who had provided information on all possible variables. A detailed description of the segmentation analysis procedure would be outside the scope of this paper. Suffice it to say that the computer programme selects the most discriminating variable, and indicates how the initial segmentation should be made. The process continues in each sub-group until no further statistical differences can be found or until the resulting sub-groups would consist of fewer than 20 respondents.

On this occasion the most important factor in determining whether a woman was in group A, B or C was found to be whether or not she had (or had had) children (Figure 1). Taking first the women without children (401, 38%), 27% belonged to group A, 39% to group B and 34% to group C. The figures for women with children (663, 62%) were 36%, 44% and 20% respectively. In other words, the figures being relative in the two groups, nulliparity increased a woman's chances to be in group C, whilst the having of children increased the likelihood of her being in groups A or B.

The second most important factor, both for nulliparous

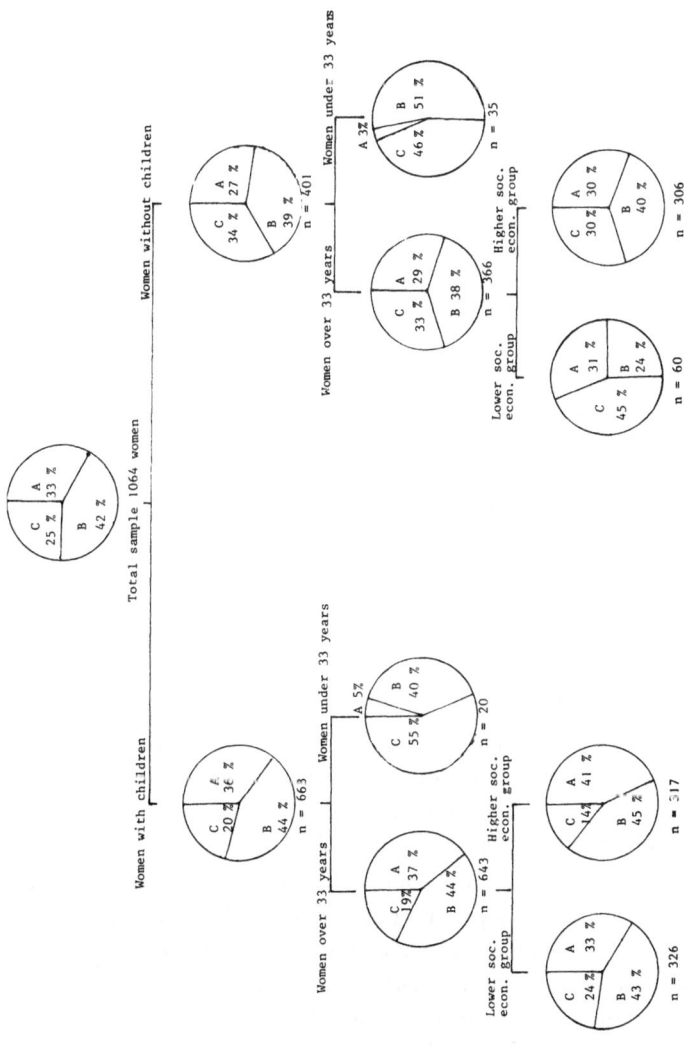

Figure 1 Results of segmentation analysis. A = symptoms related to water retention and secondarily to general uneasiness and fatigue; B = 'nervous' complaints; C = aches and pains

women and for those with children, was age. In both cases, women under 33 years of age were rarely found in group A, the group governed by D3, symptoms related to water retention, and D4, general uneasiness and fatigue. Thereafter, the profession, either of the woman herself or of her husband, became the influencing factor.

DISCUSSION

Among the facts to emerge from the French study were:

(a) 85% of the 2501 respondents had at one time or another experience of premenstrual syndrome;

(b) 77% still experienced premenstrual syndrome in one degree or another;

(c) 38% experienced premenstrual syndrome regularly every month.

These data are worth noting, especially in view of the fact that the study was conducted in a large unbiased sample, one which may be regarded as being representative of the French female population of fertile age.

The link between parity and an increased tendency to suffer premenstrual syndrome is not new, but the links between PMS and irregular menstrual cycles and prolonged menstrual bleeding seem not to have been reported before.

Turning to the statistical, heuristic, exercise carried out on the French data, the surprising emergence of three such distinct groups of women leads to the speculation that it is perhaps not *one* premenstrual syndrome with which we are dealing – but *three*. It would not be unthinkable that each of these three syndromes has its own aetiology, and, therefore, that each requires a different therapy. This might explain the variety in the ways in which women experience the premenstrual syndrome. It might also explain why some women react favourably to a given therapy, whilst others do not.

An alternative explanation could be that there is only one underlying disorder, but that environmental factors determine, in part, the way in which this is clinically expressed. It is a great pity that more explaining variables were not available for analysis. It would indeed be very interesting to conduct a similar study, similar in size and character that is, and to include for analytical purposes the endocrine profiles of the respondents. It is likely that such a study would indeed provide good insight into the cause of the premenstrual syndrome or syndromes. Unfortunately, however, it seems likely that such a study would be prohibitively expensive.

References

Bickers, W. and Wood, M. (1951). Premenstrual tension; rational treatment. *Tex. Rep. Biol. Med.*, **9**, 406

Clare, A. W. (1977). Psychological profiles of women complaining of premenstrual symptoms. *Curr. Med. Res. Opin.*, **4** (Suppl. 4), 23

Dalton, K. (1969). *The Menstrual Cycle*. (New York: Pantheon)

Dalton, K. (1977). *The Premenstrual Syndrome and Progesterone Therapy*. (London: Heinemann, and Chicago: Year Book Medical Publishers)

Dalton, K. (1980). Cyclical criminal acts in premenstrual syndrome. *Lancet*, **2**, 1070

Frank, R. T. (1931). The hormonal causes of premenstrual tension. *Arch. Neurol. Psychiatr.*, **26**, 1053

Herschberg, A. D. (1966). Données statistiques sur l'étiologie et les traitements des mastopathies prémenstruelles. *C. R. Soc. Franç. Gynéc.*, nr. 5, May 1966

International Health Foundation (1979). *The Premenstrual Syndrome.* (Brussels/Geneva: International Health Foundation)

van Keep, P. A. and Haspels, A. A. (1979). Het premenstruele syndroom, een epidemiologisch onderzoek. *J. Drug. Res.*, **4**, 568

van Keep, P. A. and Lehert, P. (1980). Le syndrome pré-menstruel; une étude épidémiologique en France. *Contracept. Fertil. Stéril.*, **8**, 775

Kessel, N. and Coppen, A. (1963). The prevalence of common menstrual symptoms. *Lancet*, **2**, 61

Lehert, P. and van Keep, P. A. (1980). La nature du syndrome prémenstruel: une classification sur la population française et recherche de variables explicatives. (Available as a manuscript from International Health Foundation, 8 avenue Don Bosco, 1150 Brussels, Belgium)

Morton, J. H., Additon, H., Addison, R. G., Hunt, L. and Sullivan, J. J. (1953). A clinical study of premenstrual tension. *Am. J. Obstet. Gynecol.*, **65**, 1182

Sutherland, H. and Stewart, I. (1965). A critical analysis of the premenstrual syndrome. *Lancet*, **1**, 1180

Wetzel, R. D., Reich, T., McLure, J. N. and Wald, J. A. (1975). Premenstrual affective syndrome and affective disorder. *Br. J. Psychiat.*, **127**, 219

Williams, W. F. and Lambert, J. M. (1966). Multivariate methods in plant ecology. *J. Ecol.*, **54**

3
Premenstrual syndrome – a holistic approach

L. DENNERSTEIN, C. SPENCER-GARDNER and
G. BURROWS

THE PREMENSTRUAL SYNDROME

Is there a specific premenstrual syndrome?

Changes in women's feelings, behaviour and social inter-actions in relation to the menstrual cycle have been observed for centuries. The term 'premenstrual tension' was introduced by Frank (1931) to describe a specific and severe syndrome of 'indescribable tension and irritability' present from 10 to 7 days preceding menstruation and relieved by the onset of menses. Israel (1938) reported that women with premenstrual tension suffered in the premenstrual fortnight 'a cyclic alteration of personality', unreasonable emotional outbursts, headache and 'nymphomania'. Later authors such as Dalton (1964) more broadly defined a premenstrual syndrome as a cluster of symp-toms, both psychological and physical, which appear episodi-cally in relation to the phases of the menstrual cycle. Dalton (1980) has emphasized that a symptom-free phase of a mini-mum of 7 days per cycle is needed to distinguish the syndrome from 'menstrual distress', a condition in which symptoms in-crease during the premenstrual week but are present through-out the cycle.

Various physical, psychological and behavioural changes have been suggested to comprise the premenstrual syndrome. The most prominent symptoms complained of by a group of women with a symptom-free phase in the menstrual cycle were irritability, swelling, depression, painful or tender breasts, tension and mood swings (Haskett *et al.*, 1980).

The incidence of the premenstrual syndrome varies depending on the definition of the syndrome used, sampling procedure and method. Many of the epidemiological studies have been based on retrospective questioning despite reports (McCance *et al.*, 1937; May, 1976) that there was no relationship between retrospective interview reporting of mood changes and that found by daily records.

Dalton (1980) reported that approximately half of all newly referred patients to a premenstrual syndrome clinic are found *not* to be suffering from premenstrual syndrome according to a definition requiring 7 symptom-free days. Haskett *et al.* (1980) rejected from their study 80% of volunteers who had claimed severe premenstrual symptoms. These results suggest that more women label their complaints as being due to a 'premenstrual syndrome' than do investigators. In addition, the use of different definitions of the syndrome or the failure to even specify the definitions used may hamper the comparison of research findings.

AETIOLOGY

Biological

A biological basis is suggested by the finding that female primates observed in the field have cyclic irritability corresponding to their fertility cycle (Janowsky *et al.*, 1966).

Mechanisms proposed include a relative deficiency of progesterone (Frank, 1931; Israel, 1938), excessive aldosterone action (Dalton, 1964), increased prolactin levels (Horrobin, 1973), decreased pyridoxine (Brush, 1979), and prostaglandin activity (Wood and Jakubowicz, 1980).

Conflicting results have been reported from studies which have compared hormone levels of premenstrual syndrome sufferers with those of controls. There is also little agreement from clinical trials based on these hypotheses. This may at least partly reflect the criteria of selection of patients for such studies.

Interestingly, most uncontrolled or single-blind studies report high rates of success no matter what the substance studied. Double-blind studies have found placebo to be very effective in the therapy of premenstrual complaints. This suggests that psychological factors probably play an important role in the aetiology of the premenstrual syndrome and therapeutic regimes.

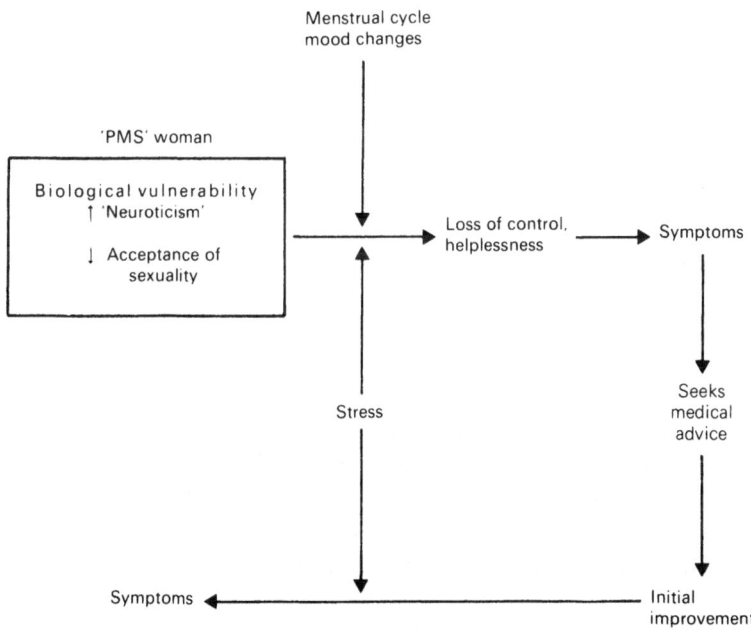

Figure 1   Factors in premenstrual tension

Psychological

There is an accumulating body of evidence relating to the possible aetiological roles of social learning (for example, of an association between menses and discomfort) and attribution by society of complaints to the menstrual cycle. The suggestion that premenstrual tension represents a rejection of femininity has not been confirmed in a recent study (Watts *et al.*, 1980), which did find that sufferers from the premenstrual syndrome had significantly raised trait anxiety and neuroticism scores and more negative attitudes to their bodies, genitals, sex and masturbation. Several studies link premenstrual tension with psychiatric ill-health. Women with emotional and sexual problems are more likely to report premenstrual complaints (Wood *et al.*, 1979). Psychiatric in-patients report significantly more severe distress on the Moos Menstrual Distress Questionnaire than do normal women (Zola *et al.*, 1979).

HYPOTHESES

It seems likely that there are some women who are unusually sensitive to endogenous hormonal changes and who present little evidence of intrapsychic or environmental stress as causative factors. Clinical experience suggests that these women form the minority of those who present with premenstrual complaints.

The biological profile of the average premenstrual syndrome sufferer suggests the following hypotheses: the woman most liable to suffer from premenstrual complaints is likely to be a vulnerable person by virtue of both biological and personality factors. High trait anxiety suggests a tendency to perceive situations as 'ego-threatening' (Shedletsky and Endler, 1974) with lowering of self-esteem or self-concept. High neuroticism scores are associated with irritability, nervousness, worry, mood changes, guilt and dissatisfaction (Tellegen, 1978). Biological vulnerability means she is likely to experience severe menstrual cycle mood fluctuations or other cyclical symptoms. This may reflect abnormalities of her hormonal milieu or of other substances, or even an individual sensitivity to normal hormone levels.

If these symptoms occur at the time of some other stress, feelings of loss of control and helplessness may be increased. As this woman has poor acceptance of her body image and sexuality, the genital organs may become the focus of fears. The woman then seeks medical advice, presenting as symptoms the menstrual-related changes which may have been exaggerated by her personality structure and inability to deal adequately with stress. Most therapies given are likely to be initially effective – especially if given with strong positive reassurance. The initial problems (i.e., 'stress' and personality factors) remain, and, if not dealt with adequately, symptomatology is likely to recur. The whole process may be exacerbated by attributional processes, such as increased society labelling of the premenstrual syndrome.

MANAGEMENT

Careful assessment is likely to prove the key to successful management. This involves delineation of the symptoms and thorough psychiatric assessment. Women suffering from major psychiatric syndromes should receive the appropriate therapy for that disorder and an appropriate explanation be given for the exacerbation of symptoms observed premenstrually. Attempts to attribute the psychiatric disorder to hormonal changes should be dissuaded. Daily rating of symptoms should then be carried out for 1 to 2 months and preferably be correlated with hormonal indicators of the menstrual cycle. This assessment will indicate the relationship of hormonal events to symptoms and, by encouraging introspection, may in itself be therapeutic.

As a result of assessment an appropriate therapy may be instituted. A group of women may be identified with problems present only in relation to specific hormonal phases of the menstrual cycle (usually premenstrual). The major type of problem varies between individuals. Breast swelling, nodularity and tenderness, headaches, mood changes and pain are among the specific problems which may be isolated to a cycle phase. Biological factors play a major role in the aetiology of these complaints, but psychological factors such as stress may make the symptoms intolerable and lead to the request for help. Therapy will depend on the type of complaint and the specific relationship with the menstrual cycle. Antiprostaglandins are effective for menstrual cramps and bromergocryptine for breast symptoms. When symptoms are oestrogen-related they may respond to a progestogen therapy throughout the month (days 5 to 25). Symptoms which correlate with the increase in progesterone in the luteal phase may respond to an oestrogen with a progestogen added monthly to induce shedding of the endometrium. Interestingly, some patients in this group have elected to have no pharmacotherapy after the assessment phase, claiming that they had learnt more about themselves and could now cope with the symptoms, for example, by reducing exposure to stress during the biologically vulnerable period or by increasing their coping repertoire.

Alternatively, the assessment may demonstrate symptoms at other phases of the menstrual cycle, with perhaps some premenstrual exacerbation. Interventions that may prove helpful for these women include those of decreasing intercurrent problems by environmental manipulation where possible, or offering treatment (of placebo and support) to those with little capacity for personality change with a strong desire for medication. Relaxation and cognitive therapy approaches, individual or group, may help these women learn techniques of coping more effectively with stress and increase their acceptance of sexuality so that the genitalia are less likely to be the focus of complaints.

The effectiveness of this management programme is currently being evaluated in an ongoing study of women with premenstrual complaints referred to the University of Melbourne, Department of Psychiatry.

References

Brush, M. G. (1979). Endocrine and other biochemical factors in the aetiology of the premenstrual syndrome. *Curr. Med. Res. Opin.*, **6** (Suppl. 5), 19

Dalton, K. (1964). *The Premenstrual Syndrome.* (London: Heinemann)

Dalton, K. (1980). Progesterone, fluid and electrolytes in premenstrual syndrome. *Br. Med. J.*, **281**, 61

Frank, R. H. T. (1931). The hormonal causes of premenstrual tension. *Arch. Neurol. Psychiatry*, **26**, 1053

Haskett, R. F., Steiner, M., Osmun, J. N. and Caroll, B. J. (1980). Severe premenstrual tension: delineation of the syndrome. *Biol. Psychiatry*, **15**, 121

Horrobin, D. F. (1973). *Prolactin: Physiology and Clinical Significance.* (Lancaster: MTP)

Israel, S. L. (1938). Premenstrual tension. *J. Am. Med. Assoc.*, **110**, 1721

Janowsky, D. S., Gorney, R. and Kelley, B. (1966). The curse – vicissitudes and variations of the female fertility cycle. *Psychosomatics*, **7**, 242

May, R. R. (1976). Mood shifts and the menstrual cycle. *J. Psychosom. Res.*, **20**, 125

McCance, R. A., Luff, M. C. and Widdowson, E. E. (1937). Physical and emotional periodicity in women. *J. Hyg. (London)*, **37**, 571

Shedletsky, R. and Endler, N. S. (1974). Anxiety: the state-trait model and the interaction model. *J. Pers.*, **42**, 511

Tellegen, A. (1978). Review of the EPI. In Buros, O. K. (ed.) *The Eighth Mental Measurements Year Book.* (New Jersey: Gryphon)

Watts, S., Dennerstein, L. and Horne, D. J. de L. (1980). The premenstrual syndrome: a psychological evaluation. *J. Affect. Disord.*, **2**, 257

Wood, C. and Jakubowicz, D. (1980). The treatment of premenstrual tension with mefenamic acid. *Br. J. Obstet. Gynaecol.*, **87**

Wood, C., Larsen, L. and Williams, R. (1979). Social and psychological factors in relation to premenstrual tension and menstrual pain. *Aust. N.Z. J. Obstet. Gynaecol.*, **19**, 111

Zola, P., Meyerson, A. T., Reznikoff, M., Thornton, J. C. and Concool, B. M. (1979). Menstrual symptomatology and psychiatric admission. *J. Psychosom. Res.*, **23**, 241

4
An appraisal of the role of progesterone in the therapy of premenstrual syndrome

G. A. SAMPSON

Progesterone is a steroid produced initially by the granulosa cells of the ovary. Small amounts are probably secreted into the centre of the follicle before the start of the LH surge, but it is unlikely that much of it gets into the general circulation due to the relatively impermeable basement membrane. Following the LH surge the follicle becomes vascularized and large amounts of progesterone and oestradiol are secreted into the ovarian vein. The combined action of oestrogen and of progesterone converts the late proliferative endometrium to the secretory one necessary for implantation of the blastocyst (Lenton and Cooke, 1974). Plasma progesterone levels rise from ovulation to the fifth postovulatory day and then plateau for 3 or 4 days before falling if conception has not occurred. Usual mid-luteal levels are considered to be above 5 ng/ml in an ovulatory cycle and above 9 ng/ml in a potentially fertile cycle (Lenton, E. A., unpublished data).

Progesterone cannot be administered orally as it passes by the portal system to the liver where it is rapidly metabolized; it has a half-life of 15 minutes. It has, therefore, to be given by rectal, vaginal or parenteral administration or by implantation into the fat of the abdominal wall. Nillius and Johansson (1971) showed that an intramuscular injection of 25 mg progesterone resulted in normal luteal phase plasma progesterone levels within 8 hours, and that 100 mg injections gave mid-pregnancy levels. These elevated levels were maintained for at least 48 hours. Progesterone 100 mg, given rectally or vaginally, produced luteal phase plasma progesterone levels, peak levels being reached within 4 hours after vaginal administration and 8 hours after rectal administration; there was then a gradual decline, reaching follicular phase levels after 24 hours. They suggest that during absorption much of the progesterone diffuses into the fatty tissue and diffuses back into the blood stream when the progesterone levels begin to fall.

Premenstrual syndrome is a global term which indicates changes in mood, behaviour and physical symptoms in relation to the menstrual cycle. Classically, there is an increase in symptoms which reach a peak in the late luteal phase and then diminish in intensity with the onset of menstruation. There are many definitions (Dalton, 1977; Rees, 1953) listing different symptoms, but these are primarily irritability, depression, breast tenderness, bloating, difficulty in concentrating and behavioural changes. The essence of any definition of premenstrual syndrome is the periodicity of the symptoms and their timing in relation to the onset of menstruation. Incidence studies suggest that over 50% of menstruating women show some cyclical changes in mood, feeling swollen, or behaviour in relation to menstruation; it is perhaps abnormal not to show such changes. We therefore have to differentiate between those who suffer from premenstrual syndrome and those who have 'normal' changes premenstrually. The question of whether premenstrual syndrome is just one extreme of a normal tendency or whether it is a clear-cut disease entity has not yet been answered. My personal definition of a 'patient' with premenstrual syndrome includes facts such as that her symptoms are marked and affect her own or other people's lives, and that she is actively seeking help.

Katharina Dalton first suggested a relationship between progesterone and premenstrual syndrome and has since written many papers and a monograph on the subject. Her initial suggestion was based on clinical observation, but since it has been possible to assay progesterone levels several workers have attempted to find a direct relationship between progesterone and premenstrual syndrome.

Bäckström and Carstensen (1974) found that in women who have mainly psychological symptoms oestrogen levels are raised and progesterone levels reduced in plasma during the week preceding menstruation as compared to a 'normal' group of women.

O'Brien et al. (1980) reported that plasma progesterone concentration is higher in women with symptoms during the postovulatory phase of the cycle and the peak progesterone concentration appears earlier.

Munday (1977) found a deficit of progesterone 8 days premenstrually in eight women with severe premenstrual syndrome; interestingly, in six of the eight women studied symptoms started more than 8 days premenstrually. In a larger study of 58 women she found lower progesterone levels in the second half of the cycle in only 30% of subjects.

Smith (1975) found the mean plasma levels of progesterone in the 7 days preceding menstruation lower in 18 patients over 24 cycles than in 11 controls over 14 cycles, the difference being statistically significant although small. Smith was impressed by the fact that there is a tremendous overlap between patient and control group levels, and also that for any given individual the presence and degree of depression in any given cycle is unrelated to the particular levels of hormone during that cycle.

In Sheffield we studied untreated and progesterone-treated cycles in five patients in a metabolic unit. Mood was assessed by the Moos Menstrual Distress Questionnaire (Moos, 1977), and weight, basal body temperature and measures of swelling and oedema were recorded daily. Daily 24 h urine samples were collected and urinary electrolytes, androsterone, etiocholanolone, dehydroepiandrosterone, 11 oxoandrosterone, 11 oxoetiocholanolone, pregnanolone, 11β-hydroxyandrosterone, 11β-hydroxyetiocholanolone, allo-pregnanediol and pregnanediol were measured. Plasma samples were assayed for progesterone and 17β-oestradiol. We found no consistent pattern of hormonal or electrolyte change when comparing untreated cycles. In two untreated cycles progesterone levels were low, reaching a peak of 8 ng/ml; in two, levels were in the upper part of the normal range and in one the luteal phase plasma progesterone rise was absent, although an apparent luteal 17β-oestradiol rise was observed (Fenoughty, 1975).

It seems at present that we have no good evidence that patients suffering from premenstrual syndrome have abnormal progesterone levels, and hormone studies offer no rational basis for progesterone therapy unless an individual patient can be shown to have progesterone deficiency.

The initial observation that there is a relationship between premenstrual syndrome and progesterone was, however, a clinical one. Dalton has used progesterone for nearly 30 years in the treatment of premenstrual syndrome. She feels failure of patients with premenstrual syndrome to respond is due either to (a) incorrect diagnosis or (b) incorrect frequency or dosage of progesterone.

Dalton suggests a dosage range from 100 mg daily to 400 mg t.d.s. by suppository or pessary with a mean of 400 mg daily; and from 50 mg on alternate days to 100 mg daily by intramuscular injection. She advises that it is wise to start a course of progesterone treatment 5 days before symptoms are expected; most patients require treatment from day 14, but there is a range from day 8 to day 28. If patients become symptom-free the dosage and duration of treatment may be reduced. Progesterone pellets can be implanted into the fat of the anterior abdominal wall, the usual dose being 5 to 12×100 mg pellets. In a series of 100 consecutive hospital patients suffering from severe premenstrual syndrome she reports that suppositories or pessaries (mean dosage 400 mg/day from day 14) were beneficial to 75 patients, injections to nine, and an implant to two patients. Fourteen patients became symptom-free with treatment and were able to stop treatment.

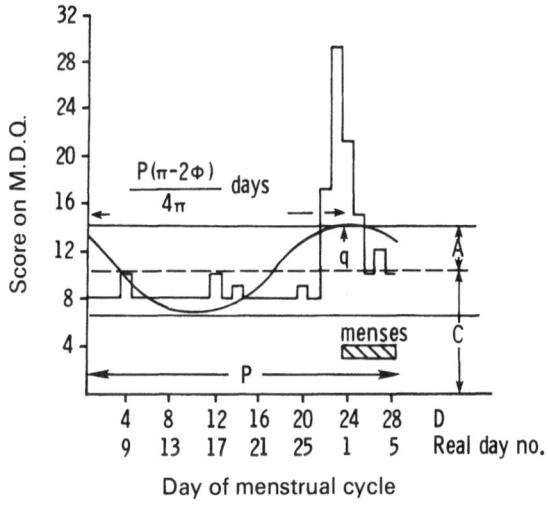

Figure 1 Data showing the negative affect scores on the Moos Menstrual Distress Questionnaire (MDQ) of one patient throughout a menstrual cycle. The least mean square fitted sine wave is also shown, and the significance of the various constants is illustrated. The sine wave is the one for which the sum of the squares of the deviations of the sine wave from the crude data is minimal

Rees (1953) reported that progesterone therapy was beneficial; Gray (1941) claimed 35 of 38 patients were greatly improved, but progesterone was given in low dosage. Smith (1975) quoted 'in our own clinic many patients have been found who seem to have derived benefits from this treatment'. In an uncontrolled study of progesterone treatment in 40 patients in the Sheffield clinic, 20 (50%) reported it helpful, 14 (35%) said it made their symptoms worse and 6 (15%) felt it produced no change.

Uncontrolled studies or reports from clinics suggest that progesterone is helpful in premenstrual syndrome. However, when reviewing the treatment of premenstrual syndrome by any therapy given in an uncontrolled study one finds impressive results. When the treatment is given in a controlled double-blind study there is usually (a) a high placebo response and (b) the active agent is usually no better than placebo. The presence of a high placebo response in a disorder of affect is not surprising and the problems in assessing response to therapy parallel those in assessing antidepressant and anxiolytic drugs.

Two double-blind studies comparing placebo and progesterone have been reported. Smith (1975) reported a study of 14 patients treated over four cycles comparing the effectiveness of four regimes: progesterone, progesterone and spironolactone, spironolactone, and placebo. Progesterone was given intramuscularly, 50 mg on alternate days from day 19. The results indicate that there were three patients who did better in progesterone months, three who did better in non-progesterone months, and eight whose results appeared to bear no relationship to the presence or absence of progesterone. They measured plasma levels of progesterone and oestrogen and found levels of hormones to be unrelated to therapeutic benefit or lack of it.

Sampson (1978) completed a double-blind controlled trial of progesterone given by suppository or pessary compared with placebo. Thirty-nine patients with a mean age of 34.7 years, 82% of whom were parous, were studied. The first phase of the trial consisted of a recorded untreated cycle, and then a 2-month crossover of placebo and progesterone 200 mg b.d. given from day 16 to 26 of a standard 28-day cycle but with the timing of dosage adjusted for cycle length. The second phase of the trial, completed by 26 patients who had already completed the first phase, was a double-blind crossover of placebo and progesterone 400 mg b.d. Symptoms were rated by both daily menstrual distress questionnaires and by retrospective reporting. On reviewing the patients' retrospective reports recorded after every cycle, when progesterone 200 mg b.d. was compared to placebo, 31% reported that progesterone was better than placebo and 43% that placebo was better than progesterone; 20% found neither helpful. When progesterone 400 mg b.d. was compared to placebo, 27% found progesterone more helpful than placebo, 35% found placebo more helpful than progesterone, and 23% reported that neither was helpful.

The Moos Menstrual Distress Questionnaire was completed daily, and the daily scores transformed into symptom scales assessing pain, concentration, behavioural change, autonomic response, water retention, negative affect, arousal and control. In order to assess a significant rise in symptoms in the premenstruum the Best Fit Sine Wave Method (Sampson and Jenner, 1977) was applied to all symptom scales (Figure 1). This gives an 'A' value for each symptom scale in each cycle which is an estimate of the amplitude of complaining in relation to menstruation. The 'q' value (acrophase) gives an indication of the timing of the symptoms in relation to the onset of menstruation and only 'A' values where the acrophase was between 210 and 330 degrees, i.e. day 23 to plus three of a 28-day cycle, were considered to be indicative of premenstrual symptoms. The presence of an 'A' indicates a significant premenstrual increase in symptoms, therefore reduction in the number of significant 'A' values in treated cycles indicates effectiveness of therapy.

Figure 2 shows the number of cycles without significant 'A' values. Non-parametric statistics (chi square) give an assessment of the difference between cycles, as shown in Table 1. Interestingly, neither progesterone- nor placebo-treated cycles were significantly different from untreated cycles in the autonomic reaction and water retention scales. Symptoms in the negative affect, behavioural change and control scales were significantly reduced by progesterone 200 mg b.d. and placebo, but there was no significant difference between the response to placebo or progesterone. Symptoms in the concentration scale were significantly improved in the first placebo cycle and by progesterone 200 mg b.d. The symptoms in the pain scale, which include headache, backache, cramps and fatigue, were significantly diminished by placebo and progesterone 200 mg b.d., but when progesterone 400 mg b.d. is compared with the second placebo cycle the placebo cycle was significantly more effective ($p < 0.01$). The results show that both progesterone and placebo are significantly effective in reducing symptoms,

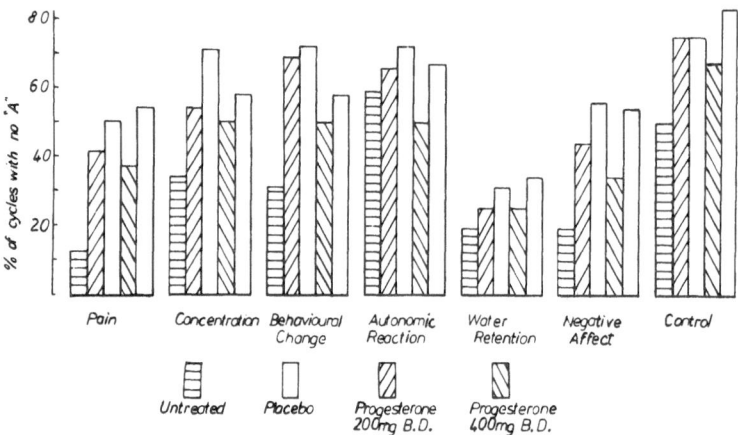

Figure 2 The percentages of untreated, progesterone-treated and placebo-treated cycles in which there is no 'A' (a measure of complaining in relation to menstruation) for each scale of the Moos Menstrual Distress Questionnaire

especially in the pain, concentration, behavioural change and negative affect scales of the Moos Menstrual Distress Questionnaire. Placebo is usually more effective, but there is not a significant difference between placebo and progesterone therapy.

The most common problem in the study was the dislike of vaginal or rectal insertion, but no patient dropped out because of this. Premenstrual spotting occurred in one treated cycle in a patient with an IUD. Four patients developed monilia, but all had had infections previously.

Table 1 Significant differences between untreated, placebo-treated and progesterone-treated cycles when comparing numbers of 'A' (a measure of complaining in relation to menstruation)

	Untreated / Progesterone 200 mg b.d.	Untreated / Progesterone 400 mg b.d.	Untreated / Placebo (i)	Untreated / Placebo (ii)	Progesterone 200 mg b.d. / Placebo (i)	Progesterone 400 mg b.d. / Placebo (ii)
Pain	●			●		●●
Concentration	●●	●●	●●			
Behavioural change	●●	●●	●●	●●		
Autonomic reaction						
Water retention						
Negative affect	●		●●	●●		
Control	●		●			

● = $p < 0.05$ ●● = $p < 0.01$

The apparent effectiveness of the placebo over progesterone 400 mg b.d. in the pain scale suggests that the progesterone in a larger dose may be increasing some of the symptoms. This apparent increase in symptoms occurs premenstrually and not with menstruation. The pain scale of the Moos Menstrual Distress Questionnaire records the following symptoms: muscle stiffness, headache, cramps (uterine or pelvic), backache, fatigue and general aches and pains. If we calculate the mean 'q' value in days for cycles with a significant 'A' for pain, i.e. the timing of the symptom peak, we find that the number of days before menstruation in the untreated cycle is 3.14 days, in the progesterone 200 mg b.d. treated cycle 1.79 days, in the first placebo cycle 2.38 days, in the second placebo cycle 1.45 days and in the progesterone 400 mg b.d. cycle 5.1 days. All these times are clearly premenstrual; the higher dose of progesterone produces symptoms earlier in the cycle and the effect does not seem to be solely explained by increased dysmenorrhoea. Pain symptoms in the untreated cycle peak 3 days before menstruation, and this confirms that our patient group had premenstrual syndrome rather than spasmodic dysmenorrhoea.

In summary, both double-blind trials found that progesterone can be effective in reducing premenstrual symptoms, but that placebo is equally effective.

These findings are in accord with Somerville's study on menstrual migraine (1972), where he found that treatment with progesterone had no effect on the migraine of four out of six patients, that it reduced the severity and duration in one patient, and that it prevented the attack in the remaining patient. Withdrawal of progesterone did not initiate migraine.

In controlled clinical trials it appears that administration of progesterone in the luteal phase is no more successful than administration of placebo. There are, however, many patients who claim that progesterone therapy has 'revolutionized' their lives. In an attempt to assess this claim I have reviewed patients in the Sheffield clinic who are of this opinion.

Patient L, aged 37, developed recurrent episodes of depression, anergia, loss of appetite, difficulty in concentrating, sleep disturbance, headaches, anxiety and bloated feeling at the age of 34 years. In the 6 months prior to the onset of symptoms she had a haemorrhoidectomy, a total dental extraction and an illness diagnosed as glandular fever. Her symptoms were so marked that she had been admitted to a psychiatric hospital on several occasions and received antidepressants, anxiolytics and ECT, with no benefit. Her menarche was at 14 years; she had regular pain-free menses and no mood changes with menstruation. She had two pregnancies, the first at 25 years resulted in a stillbirth, the second at 30 years was a full-term normal delivery. She had no pre-eclamptic toxaemia, postnatal depression or 3-day 'blues' with either pregnancy. Menstruation returned regularly after the second pregnancy and for 4 years was uneventful. There was no family history of psychiatric illness or premenstrual syndrome; she had a stable marriage, and we could find no evidence of psychological stress sufficient to induce her symptoms. The patient was eventually admitted to a metabolic unit and studied over an untreated and a progesterone-treated cycle, progesterone being given 100 mg i.m. daily from day 16 to 28. Figure 3 shows daily scores on the eight scales of the Moos Menstrual Distress Questionnaire and her plasma progesterone levels. Her behavioural change and negative affect scales were significantly improved in the treated cycle. Her fluid retention symptoms began on day 10 of the treated cycle, although they had not started until day 14 of the untreated cycle. In the second cycle there was a rise in plasma progesterone by day 8 of the cycle; there was, however, no corresponding ovulatory 17β-oestradiol peak. During progesterone therapy normal luteal phase plasma progesterone levels were maintained, but during the same time the oestrogen : progesterone ratio was consistently low. Although the plasma progesterone levels in the treated cycle appeared to reach twice the value of those in the untreated cycle, urinary pregnanediol levels remained similar in

61

both cycles, as did levels of allo-pregnanediol. Urinary pregnanolone was excreted at levels approximately twice as high during the treated cycle as during the untreated cycle.

This patient's clinical progress has been recorded over an 8-year period; the first 3 years are illustrated in Figure 4. She felt that progesterone 100 mg i.m. from day 16 to day 28 of her cycle

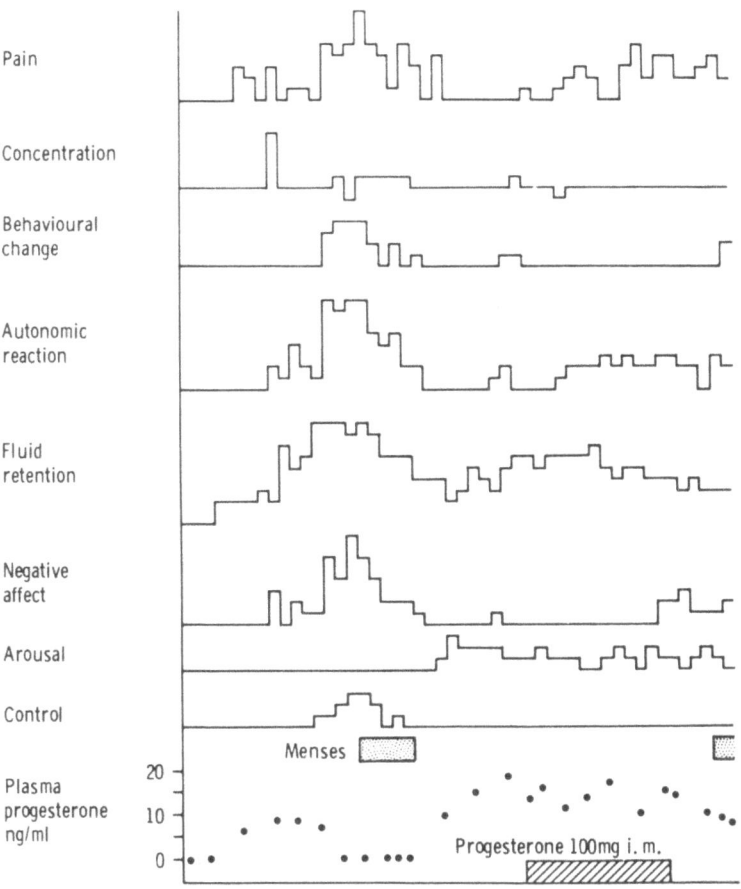

Figure 3 Daily Moos Menstrual Distress symptom scores and plasma progesterone levels in an untreated and in a progesterone-treated cycle

reduced the intensity and frequency of her symptoms, but it also altered her cycle pattern from a regular 24/26-day cycle to an irregular cycle with a longer length. She soon developed problems with heavy continuous bleeding and after 5 calendar months her therapy was altered to progesterone p.v., 1000 mg b.d., progesterone 50 mg i.m. on alternate days from day 17 to 27 of a superimposed 28-day cycle. This virtually suppressed menstruation for 8 calendar months and also reduced the number of days with symptoms. She then, with no change in therapy, began to bleed with a 26/28-day cycle and symptoms

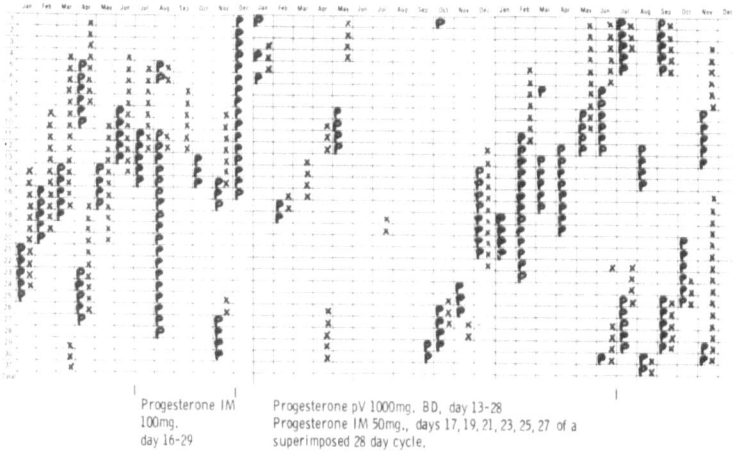

Progesterone IM
100mg.
day 16-29

Progesterone pV 1000mg. BD, day 13-28
Progesterone IM 50mg., days 17, 19, 21, 23, 25, 27 of a
superimposed 28 day cycle.

Figure 4 Chart showing menstruation (P) and symptoms (X) of one patient (L) over 3 years

recurred. However, bleeding could occur without symptoms, but after 3 months of her initial symptoms with every bleed all medication was stopped. Her cycle reverted to a 24/26-day pattern; she continued to have symptoms. After 4 untreated calendar months we gave her the contraceptive pill continuously in an attempt to suppress menstruation, and she took this pill (ethinyloestradiol 30 μg, levonorgestrel 250 μg) for 14 days.

After 3 days of treatment she became depressed and this depression lifted with the onset of bleeding 4 days after stopping the pill. After this time she had 68 days with no bleeding and no symptoms. Ultimately we suppressed the patient's menstrual cycle with 17 hydroxy-progesterone hexanoate and this has stopped both bleeding and symptoms.

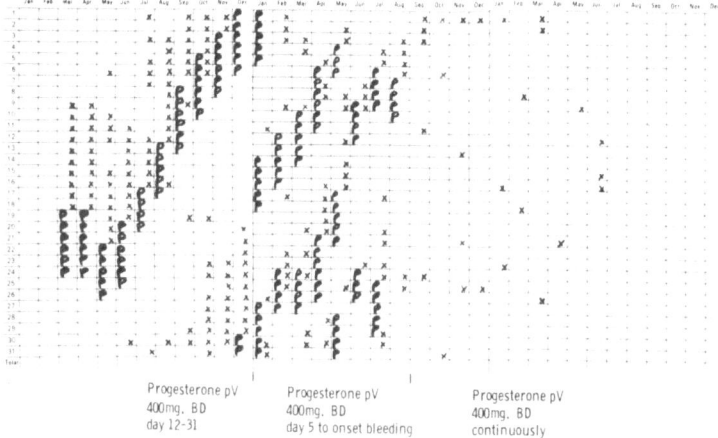

Progesterone pV
400mg, BD
day 12-31

Progesterone pV
400mg, BD
day 5 to onset bleeding

Progesterone pV
400mg, BD
continuously

Figure 5 Chart showing menstruation (P) and symptoms (X) of one patient (M) over 3 years

Progesterone therefore helped this patient's symptoms, but it also disrupted her normal cycle pattern. The more effectively her cycle was disrupted the more effectively were her symptoms controlled. She also demonstrates that premenstrual symptoms can be dissociated from bleeding. She required a high dosage of progesterone to control symptoms and alter her cycle pattern.

Patient M is 39 years old and married. Her menarche was at 13 years and she was poorly prepared for it. Her early menstruation was irregular with mild dysmenorrhoea. Her premenstrual symptoms became marked in her mid-thirties with 10 days of depression, irritability and insomnia, but her symptoms stopped with the onset of bleeding. She has had three pregnancies, two full-term normal deliveries with no postnatal depression, and a termination followed by sterilization at the age of 34 years. At first she received the standard regime of progesterone p.v. 400 mg b.d. from day 12 to day 31 of her cycle.

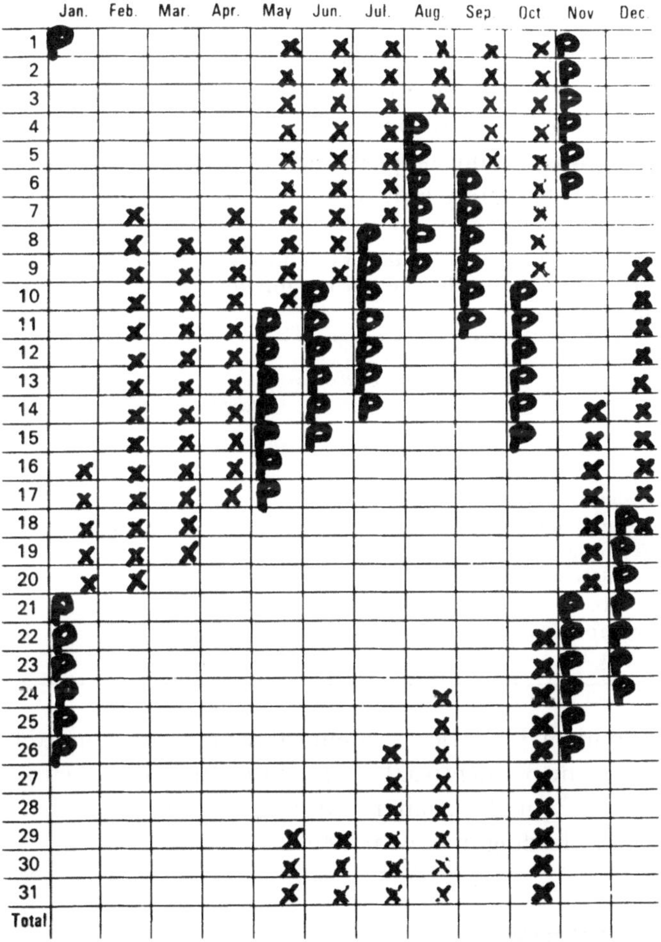

Figure 6 Chart showing menstruation (P) and symptoms (X) of one patient (T) when progesterone 400 mg noct. p.v. was given daily for 82 days from 25th January to 17th April

This did not reduce the frequency of symptoms; she reported that it reduced the intensity of her symptoms but her family did not agree that it did. An attempt to alter this patient's cycle pattern by affecting ovulation was made by giving progesterone in the follicular phase; she therefore received progesterone p.v. 400 mg b.d. from day 5 to the onset of bleeding. This regime altered her cycle length and the number of days with symptoms (Figure 5). After 4 months of this regime she failed to bleed and remained continuously on progesterone 400 mg b.d. As Table 2 shows, progesterone appears to be effective only when the normal cycle pattern is disrupted.

Table 2   The number of days of symptoms (X) and of bleeding (P) per calendar month in one patient during various indicated treatment regimes

Treatment	Number of cycles	Cycle length	'X' per calendar month	'P' per calendar month
Untreated	4	31	10	6
Progesterone p.v. 400 mg b.d. day 12–31	6	27	11	7
Progesterone p.v. 400 mg b.d. day 5 to onset of bleeding	8	14	7	14
Progesterone p.v. 400 mg b.d. continuously	—	—	3	0

In patient T we tried an identical regime; this stopped bleeding, but the premenstrual symptoms continued in their regular pattern (Figure 6), again illustrating that symptoms can occur without bleeding in some patients.

DISCUSSION

The effectiveness of progesterone in treating premenstrual symptoms should be compared with other therapies. In uncontrolled trials the effectiveness of therapy is often amazing, ranging from 91% for ammonium nitrate 1 g t.d.s. (Steiglitz and Kimble, 1949) and 90% for vitamin A 200000 units per day (Block, 1960) to a more usual 50%. Most studies using placebo find that it has at least a 50% success rate, a value which would be expected in studies treating a psychosomatic disorder.

Rees (1976) described a working model of a possible mechanism involved in the premenstrual syndrome: 'The syndrome is primarily a somatopsychic syndrome in which the physical changes are primary, but the degree of distress and disability experienced will be affected by the emotional state of the patient. If the patient suffers from a neurotic illness or has traits of personality indicative of over anxious, obsessional or hypochondriacal tendencies the degree of distress and disability associated with the premenstrual syndrome can be increased. The severity of the syndrome will be the product of the degree of changes in the internal environment and the reaction of the patient as determined by her personality, stability and emotional state.'

Any rationale for progesterone therapy for premenstrual syndrome must be to alter what Rees describes as the 'internal environment'. Although progesterone obviously can have an effect on the 'reaction of the patient', it is difficult to ascribe this to anything except a placebo effect, i.e. progesterone, although it has some sedative properties, is not an anxiolytic, analgesic or antidepressant.

The double-blind controlled trials suggest that progesterone given in the luteal phase is as effective as placebo, and this would suggest it is affecting the 'reaction of the patient' and not the 'internal environment'. Placebo is as effective and a cheaper and perhaps safer way of affecting the 'reaction of the patient'.

In the individual case studies described it appears that progesterone when it does not alter the menstrual cycle pattern is not effective. However, when the menstrual cycle pattern is disrupted there is usually, but not always, an improvement in symptoms. In such an instance I would feel that progesterone is altering 'the degree of changes in the internal environment', as described by Rees. In the same paper, Rees described a case where therapy with hydroxy-progesterone hexanoate or oral progestogens was helpful, but the most benefit was obtained with a non-virilizing androgen. Dalton has described how progesterone implants, which she finds effective, inhibit ovulation for many months and produce irregular menstruation, scanty loss, or spells of amenorrhoea lasting 6 months, i.e. progesterone is effective because it disrupts the normal cycle pattern and alters the 'internal environment'. Progesterone obviously can alter the 'internal environment'; however, one should assess if other methods of disrupting the normal cycle are not safer, cheaper and/or more reliable in their effectiveness.

We do not yet know what, if any, abnormal endocrinology is the abnormal 'internal environment' which Rees and other workers have suggested as the primary change in premenstrual syndrome upon which many secondary factors impinge. It may not necessarily be abnormal progesterone levels, and a direct elevating of progesterone levels does not alleviate symptoms. Progesterone appears to be successful when the usual menstrual cycle pattern is disrupted.

References

Bäckström, T. and Carstensen, H. (1974). Estrogen and progesterone in plasma in relation to premenstrual tension. *J. Steroid Biochem.*, **5**, 257

Block, E. (1960). The use of vitamin A in premenstrual tension. *Acta Obstet. Gynaecol. Scand.*, **39**, 586

Dalton, K. (1977). *The Premenstrual Syndrome and Progesterone Therapy*. (London: Heinemann)

Fenoughty, M. (1975). The development and application of steroid assay procedures in a study of premenstrual syndrome. *Master of Medical Science Thesis*, University of Sheffield, UK

Gray, L. A. (1941). The use of progesterone in nervous tension states. *Southern Med. J.*, **34**, 1004

Lenton, E. and Cooke, I. D. (1974). Other disorders of ovulation. *Clin. Obstet. Gynaecol.*, **1**, 313

Moos, R. H. (1977). *Menstrual Distress Questionnaire Manual*. Social Ecology Laboratory, Department of Psychiatry and Behavioral Sciences, Stamford University, California, USA

Munday, M. (1977). Hormone levels in severe premenstrual tension. *Curr. Med. Res. Opin.*, **4** (Suppl. 9), 16

Nillius, S. J. and Johansson, E. D. B. (1971). Plasma levels of progesterone after vaginal, rectal or intramuscular administration of progesterone. *Am. J. Obstet. Gynecol.*, **110**, 470

O'Brien, P. M. S., Selby,, C. and Symonds, E. M. (1980). Progesterone, fluid and electrolytes in premenstrual syndrome. *Br. Med. J.*, **280**, 1161

Rees, L. (1953). Psychosomatic aspects of the premenstrual tension syndrome. *J. Ment. Sci.*, **99**, 62

Rees, W. L. (1976). Stress, distress and disease. *Br. J. Psychiatr.*, **128**, 3

Sampson, G. A. (1979). Premenstrual syndrome: a double-blind controlled trial of progesterone and placebo. *Br. J. Psychiatr.*, **135**, 209

Sampson, G. A. and Jenner, F. A. (1977). Studies of daily recordings from the Moos Menstrual Distress Questionnaire. *Br. J. Psychiatr.*, **130**, 265

Smith, S. L. (1975). Mood and the menstrual cycle. In Sachar, E. J. (ed.) *Topics in Endocrinology*. (New York: Grune and Stratton)

Somerville, B. W. (1972). The influence of progesterone and estradiol upon migraine. *Headache*, **12**, 93

Stieglitz, E. J. and Kimble, S. T. (1949). Premenstrual intoxication. *Am. J. Med. Sci.*, **218**, 616

5
An explorative study into the clinical effects of dydrogesterone in the treatment of premenstrual syndrome

J. R. STRECKER

INTRODUCTION

From the endocrinological standpoint it seems likely that a deficiency of progesterone in relation to 17β-oestradiol during the second half of the menstrual cycle plays an important role in the aetiology of the premenstrual syndrome.

Progesterone is synthesized exclusively in the corpus luteum during the second half of the cycle, and many patients suffering premenstrual syndrome are found to have an impaired corpus luteum function. This impairment may be caused by an elevation, even a moderate one, of serum prolactin and/or prostaglandin. The regulatory effects of these hormones on corpus luteum function has been shown by several studies (Litschgi and Glatthaar, 1978; Benedek-Jaszmann and Hearn-Sturtevant, 1976; Timonen and Procopé, 1973).

If this is so, it is reasonable to theorize that progesterone supplementation by pharmacological means during the second half of the cycle may well alleviate, if not completely resolve, premenstrual complaints. Accordingly, dydrogesterone, a stereo-isomer of progesterone, was administered to a group of patients with diverse but severe premenstrual complaints. The results of this clinical investigation are presented here.

MATERIAL AND METHODS

Thirty-one patients were treated with dydrogesterone (Duphaston [R]). This stereo-isomer of progesterone has similar effects to those of progesterone, but as it does not inhibit the gonadotrophins it does not prevent ovulation. The dosage was 20 mg/day during the second half of the menstrual cycle, from day 15 to day 25.

The patients were suffering various of the broad range of symptoms usually regarded as being part of the premenstrual syndrome. In the figures which follow only the most severe problems of each patient are reported upon; in most cases, one complaint per patient. Some women were also suffering menstrual problems, such as dysmenorrhoea and hypermenorrhoea. The ages of the patients ranged from 19 to 49.

The women were treated in the Out-patients Department of the Frauenklinik of the Universität Ulm, West Germany. They were treated for a minimum of three cycles, during which time they were seen at least four times.

RESULTS

Four premenstrual symptoms were considered in this study: depression, which 35% of the women taking part in this investigation reported as being a serious problem, oedema (29%), headaches (27%) and breast tenderness (23%).

Eleven patients were suffering badly from premenstrual depression. After 3 months of treatment with 20 mg dydrogesterone per day throughout the second half of the menstrual cycle, an improvement was found in six of these patients. In four the problem remained unchanged, and in one it deteriorated (Figure 1).

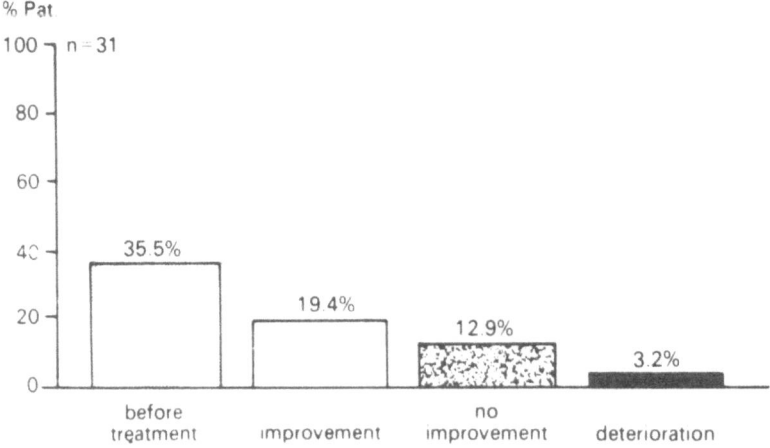

Figure 1 Premenstrual depression and the effect of therapy

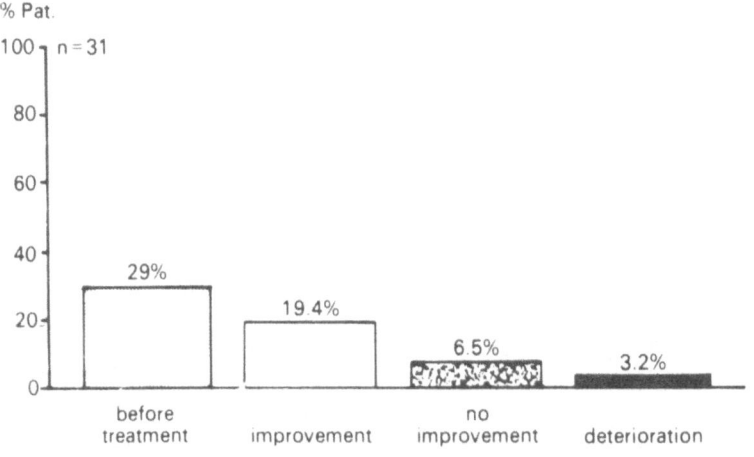

Figure 2 Premenstrual oedema and the effect of therapy

73

Nine patients (29%) complained of premenstrual oedema. After therapy, six showed an improvement. Two showed no change, and one got worse (Figure 2).

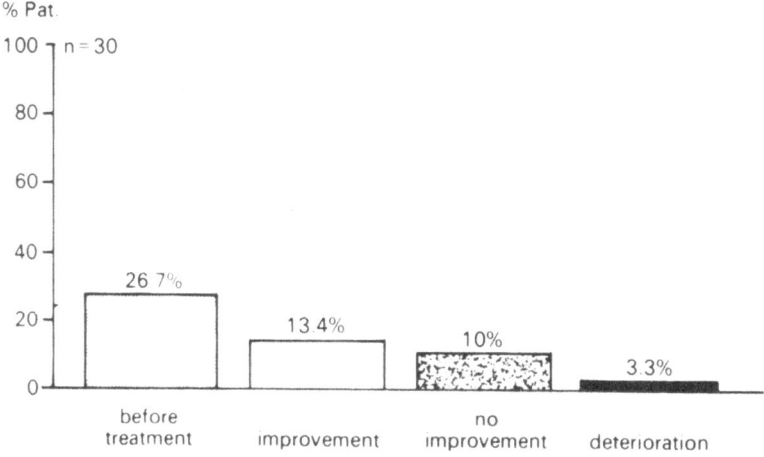

Figure 3 Premenstrual headache and the effect of therapy

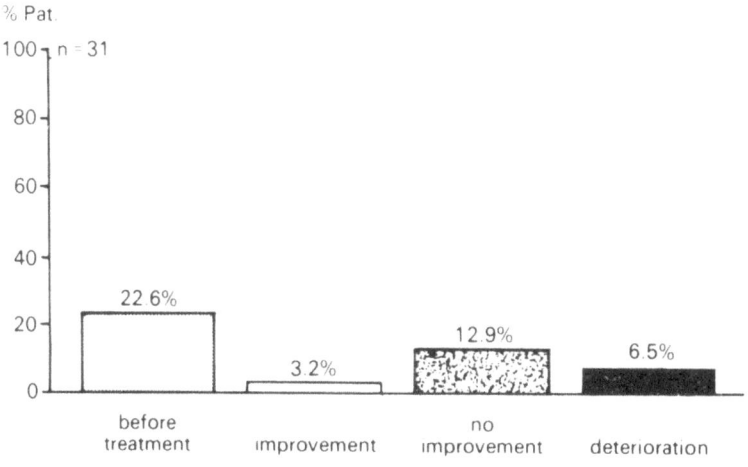

Figure 4 Premenstrual breast tenderness and the effect of therapy

Eight patients (27%) suffered serious premenstrual head-aches. Four improved with therapy, three showed no change, and one got worse (Figure 3).

Seven patients (23%) complained of premenstrual breast tenderness. Only one improved after 3 months of therapy. Four showed no change, and two got worse (Figure 4).

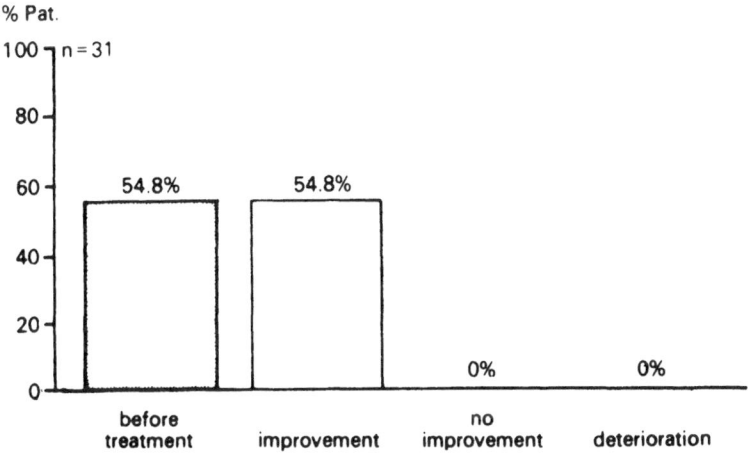

Figure 5 Hypermenorrhoea and the effect of dydrogesterone (20 mg/day in the second half of the menstrual cycle, days 15 to 25)

In addition to various premenstrual problems, 17 of the women complained of hypermenorrhoea and 13 suffered dys-menorrhoea, the two problems sometimes both occurring in the same patient. The administration of dydrogesterone for these patients' premenstrual complaints proved a very effective ther-apy for these problems too. All 17 of the women suffering hypermenorrhoea reported that this problem completely dis-appeared upon treatment with dydrogesterone (Figure 5). This was also the case in 11/13 (85%) of the women suffering dys-menorrhoea (Figure 6).

Prior to treatment, 22 of the patients in this study group

suffered irregular cycles with occasional spottings, or abnormally long cycles, most of which were anovulatory. Serum progesterone levels were low in these patients and basal body

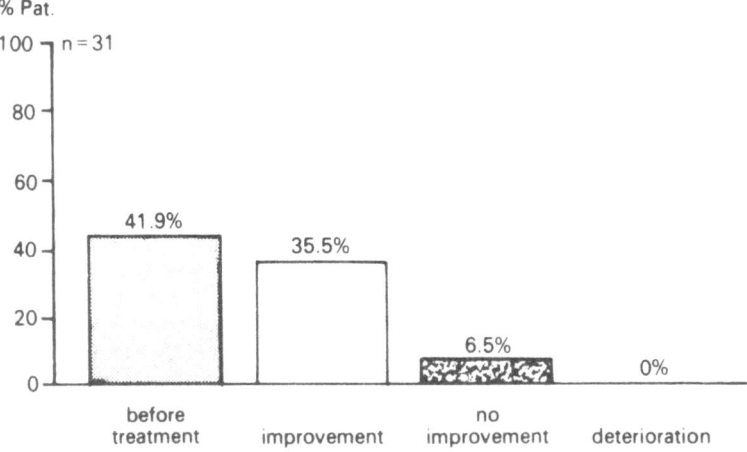

Figure 6 Dysmenorrhoea and the effect of dydrogesterone (20 mg/day in the second half of the menstrual cycle, days 15 to 25)

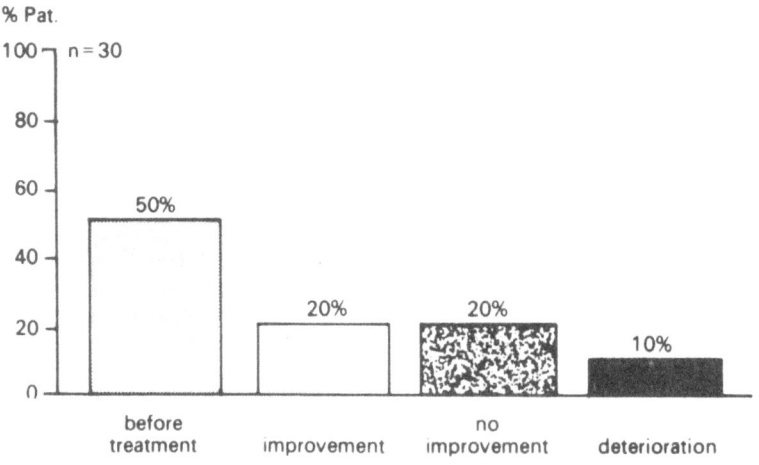

Figure 7 Effect of 20 mg/day dydrogesterone on diminished libido

temperature recordings monophasic. Treatment with dydrogesterone for these patients' premenstrual problems resulted in the 'normalization' of the cycle in 20 cases. There was no improvement in one patient and in another bleeding irregularities became worse. (As dydrogesterone does not affect basal body temperature, it may be safely given to sterility patients without fear that it will cause temperature changes which might erroneously be taken to indicate that ovulation has taken place.)

A high percentage (50%) of the women taking part in this investigation complained prior to treatment that they were experiencing diminished libido. Treatment with dydrogesterone corrected this problem in six of the women (40%).

No side-effects were seen during the 3-month course of treatment. In particular it should be mentioned that no adverse effects were seen on the gastrointestinal tract, and that no anabolic or virilizing effects occurred.

DISCUSSION

Although conducted in a small number of women, this study leads to the conclusion that patients suffering premenstrual problems are likely to find dydrogesterone of benefit in alleviating individual symptoms. In particular, it can be expected to have good results on premenstrual depression, headaches and oedema.

The study further shows dydrogesterone to be effective in the treatment of dysmenorrhoea and hypermenorrhoea, and in 'normalizing' the menstrual cycle.

It is not our intention on this occasion to make a detailed comparison of the effects of one progestational compound versus those of another, but we would just briefly mention that results similar to those given above have also been seen after the administration of the 17α-hydroxyprogesterone derivative, medroxyprogesterone acetate (Farlutal®). With a dosage of

10 mg/day, good results were seen on premenstrual oedema, depression and headaches, and also on dysmenorrhoea, hypermenorrhoea and spotting, but again the effect on premenstrual breast tenderness was limited (Table 1).

To some extent medroxyprogesterone acetate was not quite as well tolerated as dydrogesterone, some patients complaining of weariness, of lethargy, and of mild depression, though other patients, it will be remembered, found their feelings of depression alleviated by this substance.

Table 1   Effects on premenstrual symptoms of 10 mg/day medroxyprogesterone acetate administered during the second half of the premenstrual cycle. (Figures indicate number of patients)

	Before treatment	Improvement	No change	Deterioration
Breast tenderness	6	1	4	2
Depression	6	3	1	2
Dysmenorrhoea	9	6	3	0
Headache	7	3	2	2
Hypermenorrhoea	13	7	4	2
Oedema	5	3	1	1
Spotting	11	9	2	0

The generally good results reported with progestogen therapy in the second half of the menstrual cycle support the theory that a deficiency of progesterone is an important factor in the aetiology of the premenstrual syndrome. It may well be that an insufficient progesterone production by the corpus luteum during this phase of the cycle, resulting perhaps from an elevated level of prolactin and prostaglandins, contributes to, if not causes, the premenstrual syndrome. It is known that prolactin levels rapidly rise in any stress situation, and it is possible that even the mildest of psychological stresses in the days prior to menstruation is sufficient to cause a substantial rise in the prolactin level.

This paper is dedicated to Professor K. Knörr on the occasion of his 65th birthday.

References

Benedek-Jaszmann, L. J. and Hearn-Sturtevant, M. D. (1976). Premenstrual tension and functional infertility. *Lancet*, 1, 1095

Litschgi, M. and Glatthaar, E. (1978). Primäre Dysmenorrhö und Hyperprolaktinämie. *Geburtsh. u. Frauenheilk.*, **38**, 569

Timonen, S. and Procopé, B. J. (1973). The premenstrual syndrome; frequency and association of symptoms. *Ann. Chir. Gynaecol. Fenn.*, **62**, 108

6
A double-blind, placebo-controlled, multi-centre study of the efficacy of dydrogesterone (Duphaston®)

A. A. HASPELS

INTRODUCTION

The publication in recent years of a considerable number of articles on the subject of the premenstrual syndrome (PMS), both in the scientific and in the lay press, has led to an increased interest in this subject and to an improvement in our knowledge about it.

The term 'PMS' covers a wide range of psychic and somatic symptoms which occur during the post-ovulatory phase of the menstrual cycle. The most frequently mentioned are: irritability, depression, exhaustion, panic, aggression, painful or tender breasts, oedema, stomach ache, weight gain, nausea and headache.

In the past PMS was treated in a variety of ways, no single therapy emerging as the most generally accepted one.

In the late seventies, however, Taylor (1977) reported that dydrogesterone could be regarded as a safe and effective therapy for general use. In order to further examine the efficacy of this drug, a large double-blind, placebo-controlled, multi-centre study was recently conducted in Belgium, France, the United

Kingdom and The Netherlands. The data reported in the present paper are those collected in the Dutch part of this study.

MATERIALS AND METHODS

The study protocol called for the investigators to report on the efficacy of dydrogesterone and to compare this drug with placebo in women suffering at least three complaints generally regarded as being part of the premenstrual syndrome. These complaints had to occur regularly in the second half of the menstrual cycle and to disappear as soon as the menstrual bleeding began. The women had to be between 18 and 40 years of age, and the study group was to exclude women suffering from any other gynaecological disturbances, those using oral contraceptives, and those who had suffered any psychiatric illness during the two preceding years.

As laid down in the protocol, the study covered four consecutive menstrual cycles. The first, when no treatment was given, was regarded as a baseline cycle, during which information was collected about the pre-treatment PMS complaints of each patient. In the three subsequent cycles the patients were treated on a double-blind basis with dydrogesterone (Duphaston[R]) or indistinguishable placebo. Counting the first day of a menstrual bleeding as day 1, treatment began on day 12 of each cycle and continued until the first day of the next cycle. The dosage was one 10 mg tablet twice per day, i.e. 20 mg per day.

The patients were asked to carefully record the occurrence of any of the following 14 symptoms:

(a) *Psychic symptoms*
   Aggression, depression, drowsiness, exhaustion, fainting, irritability and panic.
(b) *Somatic symptoms*
   Backache, headache, nausea, oedema, painful or tender breasts, stomach ache and weight gain.

They were also asked to rate each complaint using the scale:
0 = non-existent, 1 = light, 2 = moderate, 3 = severe.

The figures relating to symptoms which were clearly premenstrual ones, in that they occurred only during the 2 weeks
before menstruation, were added together to form the patient's

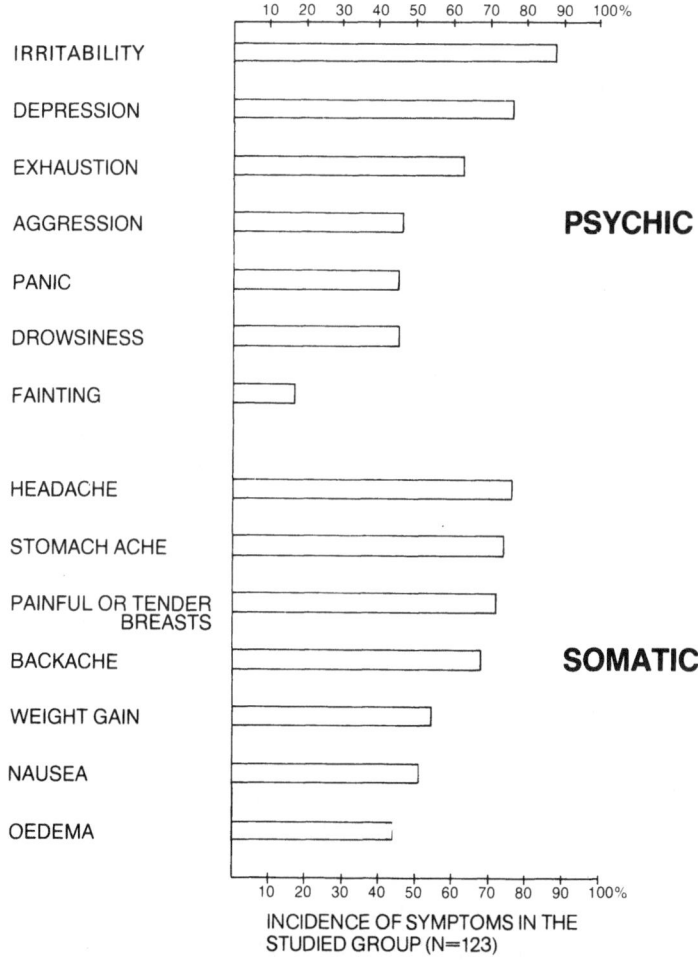

Figure 1 Incidence of PMS symptoms before treatment

'score'. The score of each patient in each cycle was thus between 0 (no symptoms at all) and 42 (the severe occurrence of all 14 symptoms).

The investigators recorded the presence and severity of the symptoms during the baseline period and again during the third treated cycle, and the difference between the two scores was taken as an indication of the efficacy of the treatment.

Sixty investigators collaborated in the Dutch study: five gynaecologists and 55 general practitioners.

Initially 150 PMS sufferers agreed to take part in this project; agreed, that is, to undergo treatment and to keep a daily diary of their symptoms for 4 months. Of these 150, 27 subsequently dropped out. The most frequently given reason was that it was difficult to comply with the request to record symptoms each day, but three patients dropped out after two treated cycles because of a lack of improvement in their symptoms. The remaining 123 women completed their course of treatment, and it is the data of these cases which form the basis of this report.

When the study was completed it was found that of the original 150 patients, 83 had received dydrogesterone, whilst 67 had received placebo. Of the 123 cases eventually available for analysis, 70 had received the active substance, whilst 53 had been given placebo.

Statistical analysis was done by means of the χ^2-test (two-sided) or Fisher test (two-sided).

RESULTS

The symptoms experienced by the 123 patients during the pre-treatment baseline menstrual cycle were:

(a) *Psychic symptoms*
Irritability 89%, depression 76%, exhaustion 63%, aggression 46%, drowsiness 45%, panic 45%, fainting 17%.

(b) *Somatic symptoms*

Headache 76%, stomach ache 74%, painful or tender breasts 72%, backache 68%, weight gain 54%, nausea 51%, oedema 44% (Figure 1).

The change in the patients' PMS after 3 months of treatment was assessed by comparing each patient's post-treatment score with her pre-treatment score, using the previously mentioned scale of 0 = non-existent, 1 = light, 2 = moderate, 3 = severe.

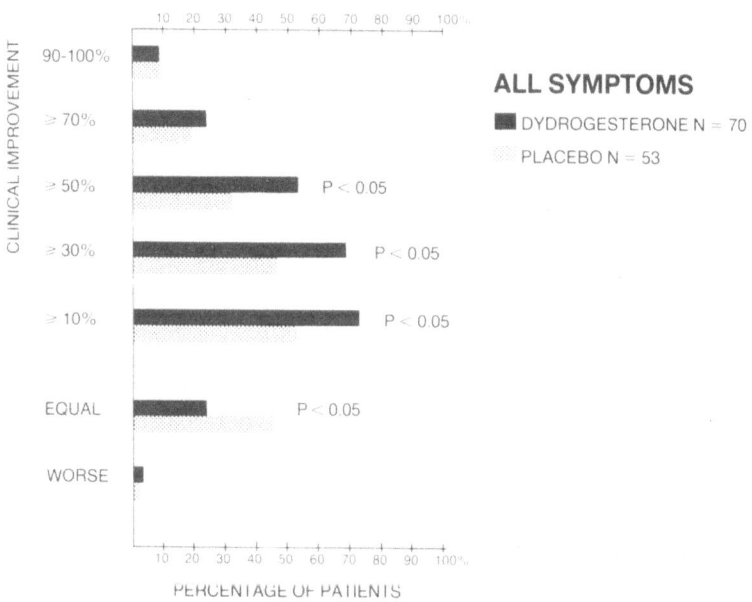

Figure 2 Degree of change in PMS after 3 months' treatment with 20 mg/day dydrogesterone or with placebo

A post-treatment score four or more points lower than the pre-treatment score indicated an improvement in the patient's PMS, a score differing by up to four points either way indicated that no change had occurred, and a score which was four or more points higher indicated that the patient's PMS had become worse. This calculation showed that an improvement had occurred in 73% of the women treated with dydrogesterone, against 53% of those in the placebo group, a statistically significant difference in favour of dydrogesterone ($p < 0.05$) (see Figure 2).

The degree of change by the third month of treatment was assessed by expressing the difference between each patient's pre- and post-treatment score as a percentage of the pre-treatment figure.

$$\text{Improvement} = \frac{\text{number of points improved}}{\text{pre-treatment score}} \times 100\%$$

This calculation revealed:

	dydro-gesterone ($n = 70$)	placebo ($n = 53$)	p (χ^2)
50–100% improvement	54%	32%	0.02
10–49% improvement	19%	21%	N S
Unchanged	24%	45%	0.02
Worsened	3%	2%	N S

As can be seen from Figure 2, the number of cases in which the PMS became worse during the treatment period was very small; it amounted to 3% in the dydrogesterone group and to 2% in the placebo group.

Using the same notation scheme, 0 = non-existent, 1 = light, 2 = moderate and 3 = severe, the effects of therapy on individual symptoms after 3 months' therapy could also be calculated. These changes could be grouped as:

(a) disappeared completely, i.e. moves from $3 \rightarrow 0$, $2 \rightarrow 0$ or $1 \rightarrow 0$;

(b) improved considerably, a move of two points from $3 \rightarrow 1$;

(c) improved slightly, a move of one point, from $3 \rightarrow 2$, or from $2 \rightarrow 1$;

(d) no change;

(e) a worsening.

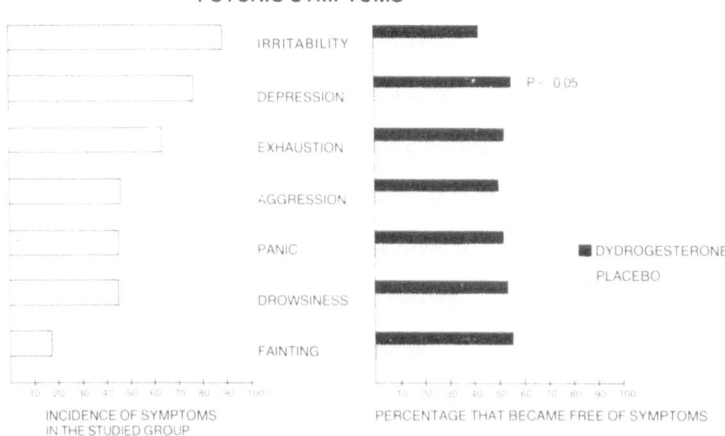

Figure 3 Percentages of psychic PMS symptoms which disappeared completely upon 3 months' treatment with 20 mg/day dydrogesterone or with placebo

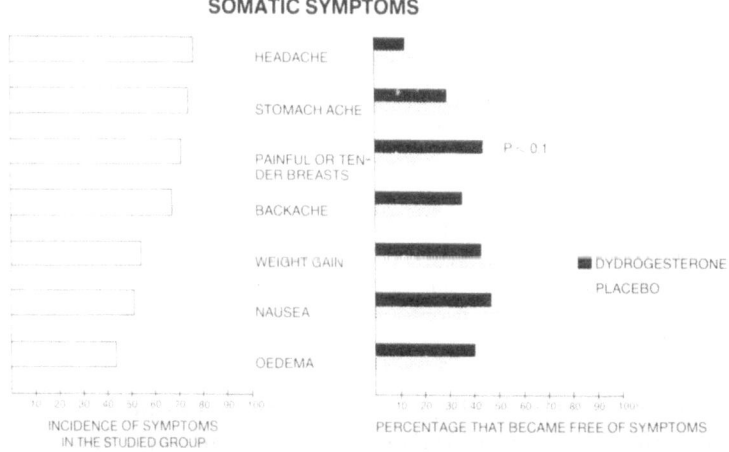

Figure 4 Percentages of somatic PMS symptoms which disappeared completely upon 3 months' treatment with 20 mg/day dydrogesterone or with placebo

87

A number of women in both treatment groups reported that individual symptoms had disappeared completely by the third month of treatment, but the effectiveness of dydrogesterone was greater than that of placebo in this respect, particularly in connection with the psychic symptoms (Table 1, Figures 3 and 4). Dydrogesterone succeeded in removing individual psychic

Table 1 PMS symptoms which disappeared completely upon 3 months' treatment with 20 mg/day dydrogesterone or with placebo

	Dydrogesterone (n = 70)		Placebo (n = 53)		P (Two-sided χ^2-test)
	Total	Symptom-free	Total	Symptom-free	
Psychic symptoms					
Irritability	64	27	44	12	0.17
Depression	55	30	38	12	0.048
Exhaustion	48	25	29	13	0.70
Aggression	32	16	25	12	0.91
Panic	31	16	24	9	0.44
Drowsiness	34	18	21	7	0.25
Fainting	11	6	10	2	0.23*
Somatic symptoms					
Headache	49	6	45	9	0.46
Stomach ache	49	14	42	15	0.61
Painful or tender breasts	51	22	38	10	0.07
Backache	46	16	38	10	0.39
Weight gain	37	16	29	15	0.66
Nausea	36	17	27	10	0.58
Oedema	30	12	24	8	0.83

*Fisher test

symptoms in at least 42% of all instances. A statistically significant difference between the two therapy groups, in favour of the active drug, emerged in this respect in connection with depression ($p < 0.05$), and a nearly statistically significant difference emerged for painful and tender breasts ($p < 0.1$).

Table 2 Percentages of moderate and severe symptoms which were cured or considerably improved, and those which were slightly improved, by 3 months' treatment with 20 mg/day dydrogesterone or placebo

	Psychic symptoms		Somatic symptoms	
	Dydro-gesterone	Placebo	Dydro-gesterone	Placebo
Cured or considerably improved symptoms (a move of two points)	55%	35%	37%	20%
Slightly improved symptoms (a move of one point)	18%	23%	26%	23%
Average number of moderate and severe symptoms per patient	2.6	2.6	3.1	3.0

A study of the *moderate* and *severe* symptoms which had disappeared or improved considerably and of those which had improved slightly, again showed the superiority of dydrogesterone, particularly in connection with the psychic symptoms (Table 2).

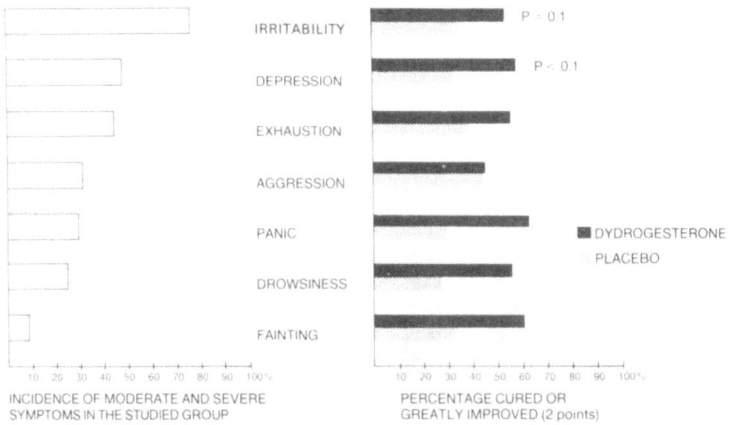

Figure 5 Percentages of moderate or severe psychic PMS symptoms which were cured or considerably improved by 3 months' treatment with 20 mg/day dydrogesterone or with placebo

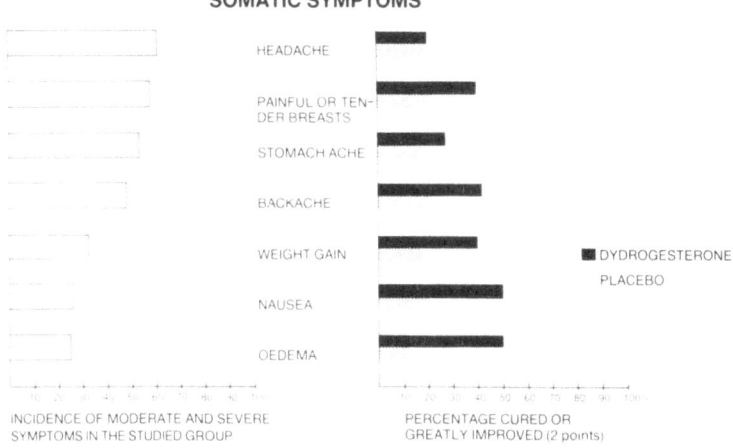

Figure 6   Percentages of moderate or severe somatic PMS symptoms which were cured or considerably improved by 3 months' treatment with 20 mg/day dydrogesterone or with placebo

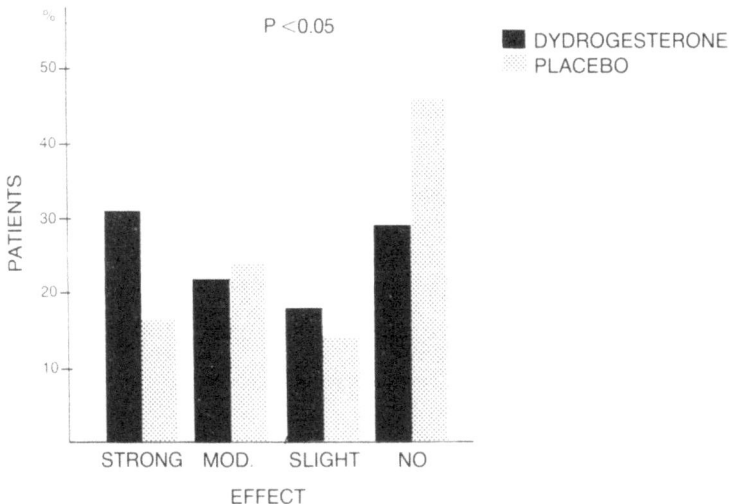

Figure 7   Patients' opinions on the efficacy of the treatment they received for their PMS problems

The number of moderate and severe symptoms which disappeared completely or which improved considerably are detailed in Table 3 and illustrated in Figures 5 and 6. The superiority of dydrogesterone over placebo reached the nearly statistically significant level in connection with irritability ($p = 0.1$) and with depression ($p < 0.1$).

Table 3   Severe or moderate PMS symptoms which were cured or considerably improved by 3 months' treatment with 20 mg/day dydrogesterone or placebo

	Dydrogesterone (n = 70)		Placebo (n = 53)		P (Two-sided χ^2-test)
	Total	Cured or considerably improved	Total	Cured or considerably improved	
Psychic symptoms					
Irritability	53	28	40	14	0.12
Depression	31	18	28	9	0.07
Exhaustion	33	18	21	8	0.46
Aggression	20	9	18	8	0.84
Panic	21	13	14	4	0.16
Drowsiness	20	11	11	3	0.37*
Fainting	5	3	6	2	0.78*
Somatic symptoms					
Headache	41	8	34	7	0.96
Painful or tender breasts	41	16	31	7	0.26
Stomach ache	33	9	33	6	0.60
Backache	33	14	27	6	0.30
Weight gain	29	13	12	2	0.23*
Nausea	18	9	14	3	0.25
Oedema	22	11	8	1	0.15*

* Fisher test

Finally, the 123 women who completed the 3-month course of treatment were asked how effective they themselves thought their treatment had been. When answering they could choose between: very effective, moderately effective, slightly effective and not effective. The replies of the 70 women treated with dydrogesterone were: very effective 31%, moderately effective 22%, slightly effective 18% and not effective 29%. The figures in the placebo group were 16%, 24%, 14% and 46% respectively. When subjected to analysis by the Wilcoxon test, this resulted in a statistically significant difference in favour of dydrogesterone ($p < 0.05$) (Figure 7).

CONCLUSIONS

On the basis of the study reported here, it is concluded that:

1. Dydrogesterone is a statistically significant better therapy than placebo for the psychic symptoms of the premenstrual syndrome.
2. It is clinically better than placebo for the treatment of the somatic PMS symptoms.
3. Moderate and severe PMS symptoms respond far better to dydrogesterone than to placebo.

Reference

Taylor, R. W. (1977). The treatment of premenstrual tension with dydrogesterone ('Duphaston'). *Curr. Med. Res. Opin.*, **4** (Suppl. 4), 35

Discussion A – between panel members

Chairman: W. H. UTIAN

Utian: I have listened very carefully to your presentations and am struck by the fact that most of you who gave a definition of the syndrome seemed to describe it in rather different terms. Does this mean in practice that you accept everyone coming to you who says that she is suffering from premenstrual symptoms as being a patient with PMS?

Dennerstein: In general at the clinic in Melbourne we accept all women for treatment who label themselves as suffering from PMS, but we define as PMS patients ourselves only those who have symptoms 7 to 10 days premenstrually and who do not have those symptoms during the rest of the cycle. Of course everyone has ups-and-downs, but we only include major changes in our list of symptoms.

Utian: So it would be correct to say that we are dealing with a syndrome consisting of a variety of symptoms that occur cyclically 7 to 10 days before menstruation and that appear to be related to ovulatory cycles, although the degree of the luteal phase involvement is in question. There appears to be a wide variety of symptoms and a wide variety in the degree of severity, but there are few, if any, specific symptoms. Is it therefore the general way in which the patient presents herself and her problem which allows us to attach the label 'PMS'?

Strecker: I am quite willing to accept the definition you have given, but does the premenstrual syndrome occur in ovulatory cycles only or does it also occur in anovulatory cycles? We have checked our patients for this and found that whilst most cycles in which the premenstrual syndrome occurs are ovulatory, there are a few exceptions.

van Keep: In our epidemiological data we found that women taking oral contraceptive pills also sometimes have premenstrual problems, albeit a bit less than in women not taking oral contraceptives. Women with an IUD, by the way, appear as a group to have more complaints than other women.

Utian: Let us now turn to the aetiology of the premenstrual syndrome. The introductory papers have mentioned a number of interesting factors that may be related to the aetiology of the syndrome. In the last 5 years we have learned that quite a number of symptoms and syndromes, some of which were previously described as being purely behavioural in causation, are tying in more and more in psycho-neuro-endocrinology. You have talked about altered hormone level ratios, but what really is leading to these altered ratios? Does anyone have information on the causal relationships beyond the altered oestrogen and progesterone ratio? What is happening at the brain level? Is anything known about the endorphin mechanism in this connection? What happens to hypothalamic functions which affect the ovarian function and, hence, the steroid profiles that have been mentioned?

Day: If I have to answer this question, I am bound to say that not much is known about all this. Professor Butt in Birmingham has done some studies in a small number of patients, about 12, looking in particular at the releasing hormone, FSH, LH and the resulting steroid profiles. As far as I know, nothing is known about the endorphin mechanism in these patients and the consequences that the changed endorphin mechanism might have.

We shall certainly learn more about this in the future. Assays are already available in some centres.

Utian: Well, the question of assays is a very difficult one, because what is measured in peripheral samples may be quite different from what happens centrally in the neuro-peptidergic pathways.

van Keep: Any effort to explain the premenstrual syndrome through endorphin changes seems to me to be pure speculation. There is a tendency nowadays to hold endorphins responsible for anything and everything that we cannot explain in other ways, and in my opinion this goes too far. If we accept a major role of the neuro-hormones in the aetiology of the premenstrual syndrome, there is a danger that we shall be tempted not to look for the best possible therapy with the means that are available now.

Haspels: In view of the high percentage of patients who react well to placebo therapy, I am still inclined to believe that there is a possibility that endorphins do play a role in the aetiology of the syndrome.

Utian: So, anything that we might be inclined to say further on this subject would, for the moment, be pure speculation. When you try to measure hormones there are so many variables. The levels may vary according to the time of the day – or night – that they are measured. They may be related to the level of stress the woman is exposed to. This goes particularly for prolactin, but also for gonadotrophins. Have patients with a premenstrual syndrome been brought into hospital and observed over a period of several days, also during their sleep? Have studies been done in which blood was drawn at regular intervals? Have the patients' endocrine profiles really been evaluated in depth?

Day: Basically the answer to your question is 'no'. No such in-depth studies have been done. It would not be very easy to persuade a patient with a premenstrual syndrome to be hospitalized for 2 or 3 weeks, and I personally am not sure that it would be justifiable to do so.

Strecker: The prolactin levels in PMS patients are usually within normal limits, but there may be pulsatile peaks in the second half of the cycle, and these peaks probably inhibit the LH production and thus the corpus luteum function. Consequently, the progesterone levels may be a little lower than normal.

Dennerstein: It was in view of the fact that hormone levels can fluctuate so much and be influenced by so many factors that we chose to do hormone assays from timed urine collections. It is a crude method, but it is an easy one. When we find an abnormal cycle we continue into the next cycle. We also continue if a woman says that she has had an unusual month as far as stress is concerned.

Strecker: I should like, if I may, to give my ideas about the aetiology of the premenstrual syndrome. One main reason for the occurrence of PMS seems to be an imbalance of the oestrogen:progesterone ratio. This is mostly caused by low serum progesterone concentrations during the second half of the menstrual cycle, which result in an insufficient corpus luteum function. As Timonen and Procopé have shown (*Ann. Chir. Gynaecol. Fenn.*, 1973, **62**, 108), a decrease of oestrogens in addition to low progesterone values increases the sensitivity of the myometrium to prostaglandins and oxytocin. This can certainly cause the symptom of uterine cramps. On the other hand, aldosterone that can be responsible for oedema and fluid retention is normally suppressed by progesterone (Taubert and Kuhl, *Med. Mschr.*, 1974, **28**, 27). Aldosterone is often found to be increased in women suffering PMS. Another important factor in the aetiology of PMS is hyperprolactinaemia. Elevated concentrations of serum prolactin cause corpus luteum insufficiency; moreover, they have a direct influence on the water and electrolyte balance (Litschgi and Glatthaar, *Geburtsh. u. Frauenheilk.*, 1978, **38**, 569). Hyperprolactinaemia quite often occurs in conjunction with elevated prostaglandin concentrations (Litschgi and Glatthaar, 1978). As I mentioned in my paper, prolactin is a hormone which is dependent on environmental factors and, especially, on the stress situations of everyday life. A certain psychic tension is easily able to produce peaks of prolactin concentrations which join the causative chain leading to PMS.

Utian: To some extent it seems to me that we are dealing with a syndrome which presents us with a 'chicken or the egg' situation. There may be a syndrome and we may find changed endocrine profiles, but we do not know which comes first. Let us now move away from the hypothetical background and devote a little time to clinical matters. I should like to ask the clinicians present how they arrive at their diagnosis? Dr Dennerstein has said that she accepts initially anyone who labels herself as being a premenstrual syndrome patient, but what, I wonder, makes you exclude a patient from this possible diagnosis?

Dennerstein: I make sure at the first interview that those who have major psychiatric disorders are excluded – those who are suffering from depressive illness, schizophrenia and anxiety states, or who have done so in the past. I also exclude after the first interview those whose doctors have labelled them as suffering from premenstrual tension but who are well aware themselves that this is not the case. To give you an example of this: I recently saw a patient whose doctor sent her in because he was certain that she had a premenstrual syndrome. At the first interview the patient told me that her problem was that she could not decide whether to continue with an affair or not, and that because of this she was becoming increasingly depressed. As this, unfortunately, happened to coincide with the premenstrual phase, her doctor diagnosed the depression as being part of a premenstrual syndrome. She couldn't tell her doctor about the affair because she was worried that he, being a male, might tell her husband. This is the type of complication that we see rather often and it is for this reason that a lengthy and good first contact is needed in order to be sure that the problem we are dealing with really is premenstrual syndrome.

Sampson: I agree with Dr Dennerstein. As I run a clinic which is quite specifically for premenstrual syndrome patients, the label has already been given to the women I see, either by the patient herself or by the doctor who has referred her to the clinic. The first thing one has to do is to take a very good history and exclude patients with psychiatric illnesses. One also has to exclude gross gynaecological abnormalities. I don't make a diagnosis at a first interview unless the case is very clear indeed. I explain to the patient what I think the premenstrual syndrome really is. Some women then immediately say 'That is not what I have got; I am in the wrong place'. Others may say that they think that's what they've got. I then give the patient a chart on which to record all symptoms for at least one menstrual cycle. We then study the chart together. I don't feed these data into the computer at a next interview, because it is usually quite easy to see from the chart when the symptoms occur. If, after this first cycle, both the patient and I are convinced that we are dealing with a premenstrual syndrome, we begin to think about therapy. If we are not sure, the patient will be asked to keep a chart for one more cycle.

Utian: Who should treat the patient then? Should it be the practising gynaecologist? Should it be an endocrinologist? A physician? A psychiatrist? Or should it simply be the person to whom the patient first presents herself? What should this person do before he can say: now I have the diagnosis and now we can start to think about treatment?

Dennerstein: This is really a good point. The situations that Dr Sampson and I have described are not really typical ones.

We have enough manpower and time and expertise and are also engaged in research. It is another thing to tell people what they should do in practice. For the majority of patients one does not need to spend very much time on hormonal evaluation. The most important thing is that one is prepared to sit and listen and accept the woman's symptoms. The doctor should then help the patient to gain insight into what is happening. Further help might not be needed. With regard to your question 'who should treat the PMS patient?' I think it should be the doctor she first calls upon.

Sampson: I have a slightly different view here. One should make a thorough assessment before any therapy is begun. This also goes for general practitioners. Most women keep records of their menstrual cycles, even if it is only the ringing of the days of their menses in a diary. They do so for all sorts of reasons. It is easy for women also to keep a record of their premenstrual difficulties. These records enable one to be sure that a problem is a premenstrual one before one begins to treat it. I really do think this very important.

Day: I have my doubts here. If you are going to give everybody a chart and ask them to keep detailed records of all their problems you risk having the general practitioners inundated with patients with all sorts of symptoms, minor ones as well as major ones. You could, in a way, attract far more than the genuine PMS sufferer.

van Keep: In our study in France we asked women if they had ever sought medical advice for their premenstrual problems. Despite the fact that so many of the women taking part in the survey had at one time or another suffered such problems (77% of the 2500 respondents were still experiencing them), less than half had ever sought medical help in this connection. Incidentally, only 38% of the 795 who had consulted a doctor had arranged to see him specifically in connection with their premenstrual problems; the others had discussed the matter with the doctor when visiting him primarily in another connection. It was interesting to see what women said when we asked them *why* they had not consulted their doctors. A high percentage, 31%, said that they had not done so because the premenstrual syndrome is a 'natural phenomenon', 44% said that their problems did not warrant it, 9% said that it was pointless to seek medical advice for such problems, 6% said that they did not like taking medicaments, and 5% said that they preferred their own remedies. Finally, somewhat strangely, 5% said that they 'would not dare' to consult a doctor about such matters.

Utian: I think that these data are interesting because in general our opinions and knowledge are based only on the women who do come and ask our advice. It is quite unusual to know the thoughts of those who do not come to consult us. I have a few more questions relating to the clinical evaluation. What does the clinician do when he sees such a patient? Is there, apart from checking the chart of symptoms, anything in particular he should do? Should he ask the woman to keep a basal body temperature record? Are there any specific blood tests to be done, or would this be a waste of time and money?

Sampson: We have heard already that most women with premenstrual syndrome have ovulatory cycles, but also that some women on the pill have PMS problems. A basal body temperature chart would not therefore be very useful. As far as blood sampling is concerned, I cannot see what conclusions could be drawn from this which would really be of benefit to the patient. Personally I avoid blood sampling in the clinic, partly because I have not found it to provide answers for the patients and partly because it does not provide answers to my research questions either.

Strecker: It is part of my routine to check whether the patient ovulates or not, but for me the basal body temperature is not the best way to find this out. I prefer to check progesterone levels in the second half of the cycle. Before this is done, however, a very careful analysis is made of the medical history of the patient.

Dennerstein: There are some patients with very unusual symptoms and I believe that in some of these cases a daily hormonal evaluation may well prove useful. Fluctuations in hormone levels can then be compared with symptoms. I have now, for example, two patients who lose their voice each month premenstrually. I would be interested to hear if anybody else has ever seen patients with this problem. You can imagine that we are most interested to see what happens endocrinologically to these patients. Hormonal profiles are also interesting in patients with menstrual migraine.

Utian: Let us now move on to another aspect: the treatment of the patient. We have heard about treatment with progesterone. We know that progesterone can be administered via different routes, and we have heard about oral progestogens and their effects. But we should also discuss bromocriptine, pyridoxine, diuretics, ovulation inhibitors, and so on. Perhaps you would give me your opinions on these different regimens?

Haspels: In my presentation earlier I told you of my experience with the progestogen, dydrogesterone. I have no experience with pyridoxine in the premenstrual syndrome. I do know, however, from my experience with the contraceptive pill and with oestrogen therapy in the post-menopause, that there may be a change in tryptophan metabolism as a result of oestrogen administration. For this reason we routinely recommend the administration of pyridoxine, 125 mg/day in the tablet-free days. My clinical impression is that this is effective. The situation might well not be the same when one is talking about premenstrual depression. If a woman is depressed it is indeed possible that this is due to a pyridoxine deficiency, and, hence, to a disturbed tryptophan metabolism, but it is most likely that depression from this cause would occur throughout the cycle, not just during the premenstrual phase. I also have the impression from the literature that any effects of pyridoxine on PMS are very close to those of placebo therapy.

Day: I can confirm that last point. In a study carried out in 70 PMS patients we found similar improvement rates with both substances.

van Keep: Jaszmann has advocated the use of bromocriptine in cases in which PMS is associated with increased prolactin levels. I think he may have a point, but we seem to have agreed that PMS should be treated by the general practitioner, and I would personally hesitate before allowing a powerful drug like bromocriptine out of the hands of a specialist.

Strecker: I agree. Also, it is rather difficult to bring increased prolactin levels to normal with bromocriptine treatment, since if one suppresses prolactin levels too far, there will also be an insufficient corpus luteum. I personally think it might be better, and less complicated, to correct the oestrogen/progesterone imbalance in PMS patients by augmenting low progesterone levels through the administration of oral progestogens.

Utian: And now a provocative question: if there is evidence that placebo therapy is in many instances as good as any other therapy, why don't we just give placebo to all patients? Why don't we restrict ourselves to the administration of TLC (tender loving care)?

Dennerstein: I would not go as far as that, but I do know that if you listen to a patient's complaints, if you explain to her what is happening and help her to accept it, you will certainly find that such psychological therapies can be extremely helpful in quite a number of cases.

Haspels: I will, of course, not deny the value of these psychologically supporting techniques, but since we all believe that an endocrine disorder is the basis of this syndrome, I am personally inclined to believe that hormone therapy might in the end be superior. I am, however, quite willing to accept that a combination of both therapies might give the best results of all.

van Keep: If it is, as our exercise with the French data tends to suggest, that there are three or more syndromes beneath the present PMS umbrella, it is likely that we shall need three or more different therapies in order to satisfactorily handle all PMS problems. The lack of adequate diagnostic techniques for PMS means that at the present time there is little alternative but to try various therapies and see how the patient reacts to them. Although some of the more powerful drugs mentioned in this discussion should clearly be used only in special situations, others, dydrogesterone for example, seem very safe and effective.

Day: I am inclined to agree with that. We have had very good results with dydrogesterone, and definitely found it to be superior to placebo. We also use bromocriptine and danazol, but would not favour these drugs being handled by the general practitioner. Some patients, it is true, may need specific anti-depressive therapy, but these may well be patients who are suffering another problem, and not PMS as such.

Utian: I think we have now covered sufficient aspects of premenstrual syndrome in this discussion between the panel members. I thank you all for your contributions and I now return the chair to Dr van Keep for a discussion in which members of the audience are invited to join.

Discussion B – between panel members and members of the audience

Chairman: P. A. VAN KEEP

van Keep: The first discussion session was devoted to the putting straight of a number of very basic points, and it was, I thought, a very well-structured discussion. The present discussion can take whichever direction you, the members of the audience, wish. We might, nevertheless, start from the same point. Are there any comments on the panel members' opinions on terminology?

K. Dalton (London, UK): There was one point which was perhaps not as strongly made as it might have been, and that is that in order to qualify as being part of the premenstrual syndrome, a complaint, besides being present during the second half of the menstrual cycle, has to be completely *absent* for at least 7 days post-menstrually. A complicating factor, and an error to my mind, arises when one uses the Moos Menstrual Distress Questionnaire in this connection. This questionnaire contains a list of symptoms, a very long list, which includes not only premenstrual symptoms but also, as its name implies, other problems which lead to menstrual distress, i.e. endometriosis, dyspareunia, chronic depression, problems arising from ovarian cysts, salpingitis, etc., problems which exist throughout the month but which get *worse* premenstrually. In my opinion, and this is particularly important when one is considering treatment, if one is talking about premenstrual syndrome, one must discard all these problems and consider solely those which exist only during the premenstrual phase, and not during the rest of the cycle. My definition of the premenstrual syndrome, therefore, is symptoms which occur regularly in the 2 weeks before menstruation, but not at all for at least 1 week after menstruation.

van Keep: Thank you. I think that is a fair comment.

L. J. Jaszmann (Bennekom, The Netherlands): The point I should like to make is a small one really, but I should like to draw attention to the fact that premenstrual symptoms sometimes occur even when there is no menstruation: in cases where a hysterectomy but not an oophorectomy has been done for instance.

Strecker: In that case I would consider the term 'premenstrual' inappropriate. A group of investigators in Belgium recently found that after hysterectomy the blood supply to the ovaries may be partially impaired (Donnez *et al.*, 1980, *Acta Endocrinol. (Kbh)*, Suppl. 234, 106). The result is an insufficient function of the corpus luteum, which might explain why these patients suffer from a 'premenstrual' syndrome.

van Keep: Would you not then expect climacteric complaints rather than PMS ones? Richards has described this phenomenon in about 70% of hysterectomized patients (*Lancet*, 1974, **2**, 983).

Strecker: The patients I mentioned were ovulating, they had a biphasic temperature curve but low progesterone levels.

Utian: The findings that Dr Strecker mentioned are in disagreement with our data from the University of Cape Town and the Case Western Reserve University in Cleveland. We looked very closely at ovarian function before, during and following hysterectomy, studying pituitary hormones and steroid profiles. We found that, although there are very interesting changes in the immediate post-operative phase, within a short space of time patients go back to full normal ovulatory function.

van Keep: Whether or not the blood supply of the ovaries – and consequently also ovarian function – is affected by hysterectomy might depend on the surgical skill of the gynaecologist.

Dalton: There may also be differences according to why the hysterectomy was done in the first place. I have found, however, that the patient who has premenstrual syndrome before hysterectomy often has the same symptoms after the operation.

van Keep: So much for hysterectomy. Let us return to the more frequently seen situation, that of the woman with complaints preceding menstruation.

M. de Senarclens (Geneva, Switzerland) : What I have missed in everything that was said is that we should try to understand the significance that such complaints have for the individual patient. If you begin to administer hormones before you have any real insight into the underlying problems you might make mistakes. Secondly, it might be interesting to see how the hormonal profiles of patients develop under psychotherapy alone.

Dennerstein: I agree with you. I personally believe that we should try very hard to understand what the symptoms mean for the individual patient. This is why I insist on a detailed assessment being made at the outset. Some people find that their complaints become tolerable once they understand what is happening. As far as your second point is concerned, a study of the hormonal correlates of psychotherapy would indeed be interesting, and it would not be a difficult thing to do.

de Senarclens: How many patients drop out during treatment? In my experience PMS patients have a tendency to change doctors. I have 'inherited' quite a number from other gynaecologists. The premenstrual syndrome does seem to be one of the most stubborn syndromes in gynaecology.

Sampson: My problem is that the patients do not drop out but keep coming to the clinic!

Dennerstein: We do not have many drop-outs either. In the beginning of our work it was different. In the early days I attempted to explain to people that their problems were largely psychologically based. Some people could not cope with this and dropped out, or changed doctors, because they really wanted a medical explanation. We are now more careful in our explanation. We explain that they are people who are, for some reason, biologically unstable during this, premenstrual, phase of their cycle; sometimes we can see from their hormonal profiles why this is the case, but in most cases we cannot.

van Keep: Perhaps we could now move on to therapy.

Dalton: I do believe in a special place for progesterone (the natural substance) – as opposed to progestogen (the synthetic) – therapy. There are progesterone receptors in the brain at the site of the hypothalamus and there is no evidence that there is any affinity between these receptors and progestogen. Progesterone has a short half-life in blood, but if you administer it by injection you may see a rise in blood levels that lasts up to 48 hours. Given in a suppository, the rise is shorter; it is never longer than 24 hours and sometimes as short as 6 or 12 hours. This means that, using this method, you have to give progesterone twice or three times a day. If you give a progestogen – whichever one – you lower the blood progesterone levels, and that makes quite a difference.

Haspels: Yet I think that there is good evidence from double-blind studies that progestogens such as dydrogesterone are very effective. I have a question for Dr Dalton. You have found a good reaction both to placebo therapy and to therapy with progesterone, but what do you do in the case of patients who do not respond to either therapy?

Dalton: As I use a very precise definition for premenstrual syndrome and treat only patients with what one might call a 'pure' premenstrual syndrome, I find initially a very high response to natural progesterone. If patients do not react to a low dose I increase the dose until they do. My success rate is near to 90%. The dose is an individually tailored one, and what I am aiming at is a long-term satisfactory result.

de Senarclens: What is the effect on the psyche of hyper-prolactinaemia?

Strecker: Many patients with prolactinomas – and consequently with high levels of serum prolactin – do not show any psychic abnormality. They may have amenorrhoea, a fertility problem, retain body fluids and electrolytes, but otherwise they feel fine. It is possible, however, that the endocrine findings are the consequence of a psychic problem, because stress increases the prolactin levels, as I mentioned in my paper.

Utian: The recent apparent escalation in prolactinoma is probably due to our increased diagnostic ability. There is another possibility, however. Stress leads to hyperprolactinaemia, via stimulation of the lactotropes. From this it could be concluded that an increase in stress in the population could feasibly lead to an increase in the incidence of prolactinoma.

van Keep: Let us look at the impact of the premenstrual syndrome on the woman's daily life.

M. Smith (Perth, Australia): Many women seek help because the premenstrual syndrome is destroying their family life, their behaviour being so bad for 1 or 2 weeks out of every 4. Should the husband not be routinely interviewed in these cases? Should we not talk to the husband and, in so doing, offer him some help so that he can support his wife? There is often a great gulf between the two partners. Often neither the woman nor her husband really understands why the woman is behaving as she is.

Dennerstein: I am glad that you have raised this point because the premenstrual syndrome really can have devastating effects on the family. I know of at least three divorces because of the hostility and aversion which existed during the premenstrual phase. I have at this moment a most difficult case in which the wife suffers a very severe premenstrual and menstrual migraine. Her psychological profile is essentially normal, which in view of the stress she is under is rather surprising. Each month she is completely incapacitated and bed-ridden for 6 days. Her two young children have to go to her in-laws, and her husband has to take time off from work to nurse her. We do see the husbands of premenstrual patients. Often we do not have to invite them because they come spontaneously with their wives, so glad are they that something might finally be done about the problem. Also, they want to tell us how bad it is for them. They also want, however, to know what they can do to help. When you ask women what their husbands have done to help them in the past, they often say that what their husbands did was not very helpful and in fact even made it worse. When you succeed in sorting out what is helpful for the individual woman you are really helping the couple.

Day: I have a similar experience. I sometimes feel too that PMS can be a manifestation of minor problems in a couple's relationship.

van Keep: Now to a somewhat wider aspect: the influence of culture as a whole on the syndrome. We could not find differences between socio-economic groups, but what about completely different cultures? Does the syndrome occur, for example, in primitive cultures?

Smith: I spent a number of years working in obstetrics and gynaecology in New Guinea. The difference between the European-type people and the local people there in this respect was very clear. As far as the local people were concerned, I never saw people presenting with premenstrual tension nor with climacteric complaints, but in the European-type people I certainly did. This may be explained by the whole cultural situation and by the differing attitudes towards menstruation. There might perhaps also be another explanation: because of the number of pregnancies which more primitive people tend to have, and more especially, because of their prolonged periods of nursing, women in these societies do not have many menstrual cycles. The question then is: what is normal, their situation or ours? It may be that, in the general scheme of things, the quick succession of menstrual cycles is abnormal and that this, as such, causes stress. There is no doubt in my mind that this stress is the major factor in the aetiology of the syndrome. We have to find out what women feel about menstruation and what in these feelings leads to the stress that induces the endocrine changes.

van Keep: Hardly any studies have been done into this, and those that have been done have mostly been undertaken in rather biased groups: medical students, psychology students, nurses, etc. Even less is known about attitudes towards menstruation in primitive societies. I wonder, however, if you are not taking it too far when you are seeking an explanation of the premenstrual syndrome in women's attitudes towards the menstrual bleeding.

A. H. Crisp (London, UK): Those who postulate psychosocial stress as a causal factor in premenstrual syndrome seem to imply that this stress occurs only in the second half of the menstrual cycle. Is this right? If so, what exactly are the stresses which occur at this time?

Sampson: I personally consider premenstrual syndrome to be a psychosomatic disorder, using the definition of Linford Rees; that is to say, the basic changes, in this case the hormonal ones, are physiological, and it is these which in a way alter the patient's vulnerability. The stresses are there all the time; it is the vulnerability which is the intrinsic factor.

Dennerstein: Attributional-type studies have demonstrated that the expectations of both men and women affect their behaviour; that is to say, if people expect to feel badly they *will* feel badly. In premenstrual syndrome, the fact that some women expect to feel badly is loaded on to the fact that they are biologically unstable at that time. They are, therefore, more likely to suffer when stresses occur at that time than when the same stresses occur during the follicular phase of the cycle or even during the ovulatory phase.

J. Laferla (Ann Arbor, USA): I am impressed by the multi-dimensional approach of this workshop. I think this approach is particularly important when one is looking at the aetiology of premenstrual syndrome. I do not think that the showing of altered progesterone levels or of the fact that progestogens eliminate premenstrual complaints, in isolation, give us much clue as to the aetiology. We really have to look at this problem in a multi-factorial way. Following on from this, I would just mention that some research which I have been doing recently may have a bearing on this subject, albeit perhaps tangentially. When looking at sexual arousal in men, we found that when coming into the laboratory for the first time to see sexually stimulating films, many subjects had a low FSH. When we administered various sorts of multi-emotion scales, the only factor which was different was the anxiety one. There is, then, a rather clear association between high anxiety and low FSH. It may be that studies looking at the effects of stress could well be useful in the study of premenstrual syndrome. One last point, and this is in connection with the comments about the effect of premenstrual syndrome on family life. A colleague of mine in Rochester, New York, has recently made a study of alcoholism in young women, and found a very striking correlation between young female alcoholism and premenstrual distress. I am not suggesting that premenstrual syndrome causes alcoholism, but it may be that there are factors at work which influence both.

van Keep: Jaszmann and I once presumed that the process of symptom formation in the premenstrual syndrome, in dysmenorrhoea and in climacteric complaints must take place along similar lines; in all three instances there is a somatic problem and a psychic problem, and we presumed that these two potentiated one another. However, when we looked at women over 50 and recorded the incidence of earlier premenstrual problems and dysmenorrhoea, and of climacteric complaints, we found that whilst there was indeed a strong correlation between the premenstrual syndrome and dysmenorrhoea, there was none at all between these and climacteric complaints. We concluded from this that the mechanisms of symptom formation must be quite different (van Keep and Jaszmann, *Geburtsh. u. Frauenheilk.*, 1973, **8,** 669).

Dennerstein: We too found, using psychological rating scales, that PMS patients and climacteric patients are very different. The patients with climacteric problems were within the normal range of the Eysenck Personality Inventory ratings in neuroticism, extraversion, anxiety and depression, whereas the PMS patients were certainly not.

Dalton: In my experience women with premenstrual syndrome tend to have less climacteric problems. My explanation for this is that women with a premenstrual syndrome have a high oestrogen production during their menstruating years, so high that it upsets the oestrogen:progesterone ratio and leads to PMS problems. However, when these women approach the menopause their high oestrogen levels protect them to a large extent from climacteric problems.

van Keep: You might also consider this, rather sexist and not too seriously offered, explanation: to some extent women might suffer premenstrual problems because they resent having menstruation, and, by the same token, those who resent losing their fertility may suffer climacteric problems. However, whichever explanation might be correct, the hormonal one or the psychological one, we found no relation at all between the two syndromes.

Strecker: I am coming back to Dr Laferla's remark on low FSH and anxiety being correlated in men: if women are suffering from stress in the *first* half of their cycle this will lead to an increase in serum prolactin levels, which, in turn, will lead to decrease of gonadotrophins. This low FSH and LH might impair follicle growth and corpus luteum formation, and this could indeed lead to premenstrual problems.

van Keep: We shall have to stop this discussion soon. Is there a last question please?

Utian: Since you brought the matter up yourself, I should like to ask whether we are in fact dealing with one syndrome or with several.

Haspels: Apart from the evidence presented by Dr van Keep, I feel that the diversity of the complaints and the different reactions of patients to therapy suggest that we may indeed be dealing with different syndromes. It would be very helpful if these syndromes could be identified.

Dennerstein: I certainly know that women respond variously to treatment. I do not know whether or not I have to conclude from this that there are different syndromes, but it certainly strengthens my view that there should be an individual assessment and approach to management in each case.

Day: I would obviously like it if the complaints would break down into a few clusters, each with a different aetiology and requiring different treatment, but I am not sure that the data presented provide us with the answer.

Sampson: My work shows that certain symptoms do respond differently. I could, therefore, support the theory that there are different syndromes, but this subject needs further study.

Strecker: The term 'syndrome' is often used when a group of individual symptoms is ill-defined and vague.

van Keep: For me a 'syndrome' is a group of symptoms with a common cause. When reporting our findings and presenting the theory of there being several syndromes instead of just one, we entitled our paper 'A statistical exercise'. The clusters of symptoms were proposed not by the statistical analysis but by ourselves. What the subsequent analysis did was to show that our thoughts, based on clinical experience, were indeed logical. Considering the costs involved, a repetition of this exercise including endocrine profiles as explaining variables is not really justified. Nevertheless, the concept resulting from our exercise is attractive because it may explain why some women react to a given therapy whilst others do not. It is clear that further work is needed before one will be able to say exactly which symptoms of the premenstrual syndrome in which women will react to which therapies. At present we have to find the best therapy for an individual patient by trial and error, though our knowledge, particularly through well-controlled clinical studies, is increasing all the time. Common sense and, above all, an open mind for our individual patient's problems and needs, remain important factors in the handling of the PMS patient.

Thank you all for your contributions to this workshop.

Index

aetiology 11–26, 44–6, 94, 96, 112
  biological 44, 45, 48
  PMS model 21, 22
  psychological factors 45
alcoholism 113
aldosterone
  antinatriuretic 18
  inhibitor 24, 25
  levels and PMS 17, 18, 44
  and progesterone suppression 96
allergy, steroid 20
allopregnanediol 54
amenorrhoea 19
ammonium nitrate 67
androsterone 54
angiotensin 17, 18
antigonadotropin, PMS
    treatment 25
antiprostaglandins 48
arousal 62
  and FSH 112
autonomic reaction 62
  placebo and progesterone
    effects 58, 59

basal body temperature 53, 77,
    100
behaviour changes 61
  placebo and progesterone
    effects 58, 59
breast symptoms 18, 23, 72, 78
  premenstrual and
    dydrogesterone 74, 75

bromocriptine 18, 48, 103
  effects 25
  and prolactin 102

children and PMS 36, 38
climacteric
  and hysterectomy 16
  and PMS 106
  and skin problems 37
concentration 62
  placebo and progesterone
    effects 58, 59
corpus luteum
  control 114
  insufficiency 96
    and hysterectomy 106

danazol, PMS treatment 25
dehydroepiandrosterone 54
depression 61, 72
  and medroxyprogesterone
    acetate 78
  premenstrual and
    dydrogesterone 72, 73,
    83–92
  and pyridoxine deficiency 101
dopamine 23
dydrogesterone 24, 101
  multi-centre study 81–92
  PMS effects 71–8
  and psychic symptoms 84–7
  safety 81
  somatic symptoms 85–7

dydrogesterone (continued)
  symptom disappearance 88
  symptom improvement 89–91
  treatment assessment by
    patients 90–2
dysmenorrhoea
  dydrogesterone effects 76, 77
  and medroxyprogesterone
    acetate 78
  and PMS 113

endorphins 94, 95
etiocholanolone 54
Eysenck Personality
  Inventory 113

fluid retention 23, 24, 57, 62, 96
  incidence and PMS 36–40
  placebo and progesterone
    effects 58, 59
follicle stimulating hormone
  (FSH) 94, 114
  and anxiety in men 114
  and arousal 112
  plasma levels in PMS 15, 21
  release and danazol 25
FSH see follicle stimulating hormone

galactorrhoea 20

headache 72
  and medroxyprogesterone
    acetate 78
  premenstrual and
    dydrogesterone 74, 75
hormones
  changes in menstrual cycle 11
  sensitivity to changes in 46, 47
  husband, role in PMS 109, 110
11β-hydroxyandrosterone 54
11β-hydroxyetiocholanolone 54
17-hydroxyprogesterone
    hexanoate 68
  and menstrual cycle
    suppression 64

hyperinsulinism 20
hypermenorrhoea
  and dydrogesterone 75, 77
  and medroxyprogesterone
    acetate 78
hyperprolactinaemia 96, 97
  effects of 109
  and LHRH response 20
  and menstrual cycle 19
hypoglycaemia 20
hysterectomy
  and climacteric complaints 106
  and mood changes 12
  and ovarian function 106, 107
  and premenstrual
    symptoms 106

intrauterine devices (IUD) 58
  and premenstrual complaints 94

LH see luteinizing hormone
LHRH see luteinizing hormone
  releasing hormone
libido, dydrogesterone effects 76,
    77
luteal phase, shortened 19
luteinizing hormone (LH) 94, 114
  plasma levels and PMS 15, 22
  surge 22, 51
  and danazol 25
luteinizing hormone-releasing
    hormone (LHRH)
  response in
    hyperprolactinaemia 20

mastalgia 25
mastodynia 18, 25
medroxyprogesterone acetate 77
  and premenstrual symptoms 77,
    78
  tolerance 78
menstrual cycle
  asynchronous 22
  complaints 46
  length and PMS 36

menstrual cycle (*continued*)
  length and prolactin 18, 19
  and progesterone levels 51
  recording 99
  regularity and PMS 36
  suppression 63, 64
  and symptoms in progesterone
    therapy 63–5
menstrual distress 43
migraine, menstrual 60
  and progesterone 60
monoamine oxidase inhibition and
  PMS 26
mood assessment 53
Moos Menstrual Distress
  Questionnaire 46, 53, 57
  case histories 61–6
  deficiencies 105
  pain scale 60
myometrium, hormone
  sensitivity 96

negative affect 55, 58, 62
neuroticism 13, 46
  incidence and PMS 36–40
noradrenaline 23
nymphomania 43

oedema 53, 72, 96
  dydrogesterone effects 72–4
  and medroxyprogesterone
    acetate 78
oestradiol 54
  plasma levels and PMS 14–17
oestrogen 53
  and tension 23
oral contraceptives
  and menstruation
    suppression 63
  and premenstrual
    problems 94, 100
ovarian function and
  hysterectomy 107
11-oxoandrosterone 54

11-oxoetiocholanolone 54
oxytocin 96

pain
  assessment 60, 62
  incidence 34–40
  placebo and progesterone
    effects 58, 59
  placebo effect 12, 26, 45, 56, 67,
    95, 102
  dydrogesterone
    comparison 84–92
    effect on symptoms 85–91
  progesterone comparison 56–60
PMS *see* premenstrual syndrome
pregnanediol 54
pregnanolone 54
premenstrual spotting 58
premenstrual symptoms
  incidence 34, 35, 40
  and problems 34
premenstrual syndrome (PMS)
  aetiology 11–26, 44–6, 48, 94,
    96, 112
  climacteric problems 113
  definition 31, 46
  diagnosis 93, 97, 103
  differing responses 115
  dydrogesterone effects 71–8,
    81–92
  effects on family 110, 112
  endocrinopathy 8
  incidence 13, 32–5, 44
  management 47–9
  and medroxyprogesterone
    acetate 77, 78
  neuroticism correlation 13
  in New Guinea natives 110, 111
  numbers consulting doctor 99,
    100
  ovarian steroids and 14–17
  placebo effects 12, 26, 45,
    56–60, 67, 84–92
  predisposing factors 36
  and progesterone therapy 51–68

premenstrual syndrome (PMS)
(continued)
scoring 46, 53, 55-7
somatopsychic 67
study designs 33-6, 95
symptom clusters 114, 115
and symptoms 33, 34, 52, 81,
93, 110
disappearance 88
somatic 81-90
psychic 82-9
premenstrual tension 12, 43
factors 45
and psychiatric health 46
progesterone see also progesterone
treatment
-aldosterone ratio 17
CNS accumulation 23
and migraine 60
mode of action 24
-oestrogen ratio 14, 15, 21, 53
71, 94, 96
mechanisms of altered 22
plasma levels 51, 101
effects of 23
and menstrual cycle 62
and PMS 14-17, 19, 44
supplementation 71-8
synthesis 71
progesterone treatment 101
administration 51, 52, 58
and blood levels 108
case histories 61-6
and cycle pattern 63, 64
dose 57-60
implanted 54, 68
intramuscular 56
and menstrual cycle
disruption 68
placebo comparison 56-60
regimes and effects 66
role in PMS therapy 51-68
and effectiveness 55
suppositories 54-6
and symptoms 64, 65

after 3 years 63
progestogen therapy 48, 108
and progesterone blood
levels 108
prolactin
effects and PMS 19-22
levels and PMS 45, 96
-progesterone levels and
PMS 19
pulsatile release 18, 96
role in PMS 51-68
and steroidogenesis 22
and stress 78, 97
suppression 102
prolactinoma 109
prostaglandins 96
activity and PMS 45
psychiatric disorders 46, 47
psychic symptoms and
dydrogesterone
therapy 83-92
psychosomatic disorder 67, 111
psychotherapy 107
pyridoxine deficiency 101, 102

renin–angiotensin system 17, 18

segmentation analysis 38, 39
serotonin 23
skin problems
and age 37
incidence and PMS 36-40
somatic symptoms and
dydrogesterone
therapy 83-92
spironolactone
anti-androsterone and PMS 24,
25
spotting and medroxyprogesterone
acetate 78
steroids, gonadal and CNS
accumulation 23
stress 13, 78, 97, 109
psychosocial 111

tension incidence and PMS 36–40
treatment 48, 49, 101 *see also*
    progesterone, placebo
aldosterone inhibition 24, 25
compliance 107
dydrogesterone 71–8, 81–92
mode of action 24–6
progesterone 51–68
progestogens 24
pyridoxine 20, 21, 26

tryptophan metabolism 101

uterine cramps 96

vitamin A 67
vitamin B_6
    co-enzyme 20
    deficiency and PMS 20, 21, 25,
      43
voice, loss of 101